Healing Muscle Pain

Healing Muscle Pain

Tools, Techniques, and Tips
to Bring Your Muscles
Back to Health

Elisabeth Aaslid

with Kate A. Schultz, P.T.

John Wiley & Sons, Inc.
New York • Chichester • Weinheim • Brisbane • Singapore • Toronto

Published by John Wiley & Sons, Inc.
Published simultaneously in Canada

This publication is designed to provide accurate and authoritative information in regard to the subject matter covered. It is sold with the understanding that the publisher is not engaged in rendering professional services. If professional advice or other expert assistance is required, the services of a competent professional person should be sought.

Library of Congress Cataloging-in-Publication Data:

Aaslid, Elisabeth
    Healing muscle pain : tools, techniques, and tips to bring your muscles back to health / Elisabeth Aaslid with Kate A. Schultz.
      p. cm.
    Includes bibliographical references and index.
    ISBN 0-471-37891-7 (pbk. : alk. paper)
    1. Myalgia—Popular works.   I. Schultz, Kate A. II. Title.
  RC925.5.A25 2001
  616.7′4—dc21   00-036842

Printed in the United States of America

10 9 8 7 6 5 4 3 2 1

To
Ive and Vilde

Contents

Preface

Like most of us, for years I suffered from a variety of muscle aches and pains that my body had accumulated over my lifetime. I was treated by excellent health care professionals. However, when my treatment ended, my old problems returned. I could not possibly afford all these treatments. But without them, it seemed as if my body retreated to a state of pain and discomfort. There were, however, no obvious medical reasons for this.

I developed a need for a much deeper understanding of what was happening to me and also to my children, friends, and family members, who all were struggling with different forms of muscle pain.

I started my quest for knowledge by trying to read the classic medical text *Gray's Anatomy*. I cried with frustration over all the complicated anatomical terms I couldn't make sense of, because I was now desperate to know. My search led me to the library and to university medical school bookstores. I bought books, I borrowed books, I read and read and read. It took me a long time, and I often lost heart and felt that there was too much for me to ever understand. But I was stubborn, and eventually my perseverance paid off. As I read, I slowly came to see how I was creating my own pain daily, moment by moment, out of ignorance and unawareness of how the muscles and joints work together in my body. I found the reasons for my pain—along with guidance for healing it—in the books. It was all perfectly logical! And this voyage of discovery taught me the most important truth of all: The path to recovery lay through learning about my body and, most importantly, my body belonged to me and I had a right to treat it as mine.

This book is my effort to pass on the knowledge that has helped me so much with the discovery of how and why your aches and pains come to exist and how you can relieve and restore your muscles to health.

Acknowledgments

So many people have contributed to this book that listing everyone would fill a chapter, but I would like to extend special thanks to Ive Aaslid, Nancy T. Reynolds, and Paula Lowe; my editor, Betsy Thorpe; my medical editor, Wolfgang Brolley, RPT; and all the wonderful friends, family members, and professional associates who helped me through the writing of this book.

In addition, I would like to thank physical therapist Kate A. Schultz and massage therapist Mimi Polvino. Kate has provided invaluable professional support while working as a collaborator on this book.

Mimi Polvino, LMP, has generously shared her knowledge and experience gleaned from many years of working with dancers, athletes, and others who have suffered soft-tissue trauma. I am especially grateful for her inspiration and persistent belief in the ability of the body's tissue to heal itself when circulation is restored.

Last, I want to thank my illustrator, Susan I. Jessup, for her work. She stepped in at the last minute when the other illustrator fell ill, adding late hours to her full-time job as a technical illustrator.

Healing Muscle Pain

Part One

CHAPTER 1

Healing Muscle Pain

Our muscles are designed to be flexible, strong, and smooth, with the ability to contract and relax painlessly. After we have suffered long-term or repeated muscle pain, however, we can easily forget how our muscles are supposed to feel. In fact, muscle pain tends to become such a normal part of our everyday lives that we seldom try to treat it until we are forced to quit working or engaging in our favorite activities. Yet much of this muscle pain is unnecessary and its consequences avoidable. Caring for our muscles and relieving their pain can be easier than we first assume. We can restore well-being and health, first of all by eliminating the factors that cause the pain once we learn to recognize these. Second, just as we are taught to brush our teeth to avoid tooth decay, we can learn some simple techniques to treat our muscles in order to both relieve and prevent muscle pain.

Understanding the factors that influence the health of our muscles and contribute to pain is as important as knowing how to treat and relieve the pain. In an ideal world, we could count on our doctors and other care providers to explain such things to us. More often, however, we leave their offices with at least as many unanswered questions as we came in with.

One reason why it is hard to get answers to questions about muscle pain is that many of the answers are yet to be found. Although medical research has yielded much knowledge about what leads to pain in the muscles, many unknowns still exist. Contrary to what most people believe, even the most widely experienced pain of all—exercise soreness—has not been fully explained. Muscle cramps, spasms, stiff neck, and many other common ailments are on the long list of everyday muscular conditions for which medical research still cannot provide clear answers.

The reality, that there are too many contradictory factors to fully explain muscle pain, is certainly not the fault of doctors. But because of what is not known, the medical profession has fallen into the habit of saying nothing at all to patients about their muscles. Most people, therefore, know very little about how their muscles actually work, what contributes to pain, and what can be done to relieve and prevent it.

As laypeople, we need not concern ourselves with the complex questions of medical research; the knowledge we need in order to care for our muscles and solve our pain problems is much less complicated. But we do need to know some basics. Doctors, physical therapists, and massage therapists have a thorough understanding of the basic functions of the muscles in the body and the processes that most affect muscle health. In order to help the medical professionals heal us—and in order to heal ourselves—we also need to know these fundamentals. Without this understanding, healing is a difficult and often aimless process.

What This Book Will Give You

This book will help you to better understand your muscle pain, and guide you on the path to overcoming rather than being defeated by it. In addition to grounding you in the basics of how our muscular and related systems work (and don't work), the book will teach you how to locate muscles in your body, how to experience them moving, and how to treat and relieve key muscles in your body. You will learn that just as our posture and unconscious movements over the course of a day can create our muscle pain, it is during our day that we must make the changes that will lead to healing. Throughout the book you'll find many boxes containing exercises designed to jumpstart the healing process and give you quick relief from your muscle pain and tightness whenever it appears—anytime, anywhere during your day. You can use these in combination with the longer-term stretching and strengthening exercises to put you on the road to fast and permanent muscle health.

How to Use This Book

The book is organized into two sections. The first section provides you with the knowledge to understand what is going on in your muscular system. The second section presents you with the tools to apply that knowledge.

The book is organized sequentially, so that with each chapter you read, you will be adding a new layer of information to your understanding. However, if your concern is to relieve a specific, distracting pain first, it is okay to start by going directly to Chapter 8 and consulting the step-by-step guide. It will direct you to the specific chapter that can help you develop and work through a strategy for resolving your pain. Here is a list of the steps and the chapters in which they're discussed:

Step 1: Find Your Key Muscle. Attempt to identify and locate the muscle that's causing the problem. See Chapters 8 and 9.

Step 2: Get to Know Your Key Muscle. Learn what the muscle does (its job) and what most commonly stresses it. See Chapter 9.

Step 3: Test Your Key Muscle. Check out and analyze the condition of your painful muscle as well as related muscles that might contribute to your pain. See Chapter 11.

Step 4: Start the Healing Process. Choose from among different pain-relieving and healing techniques the one that suits your needs the best. See Chapter 5.

Step 5: Stretch and Strengthen Your Key Muscle. Carefully exercise, stretch, and strengthen the muscle back to health. See Chapters 12 and 13.

Step 6: Be Mindful of Your Muscles During the Day. With the knowledge you've gained, you can learn to give relief to your pained muscles during the day as tightness and pain appear, catch problems before they start, and take proactive steps to avoid generating new ones. See Chapter 4.

Step 7: See the Bigger Picture of Your Pain. Identify and treat the other muscles that work with and impact your problem muscle. See Chapters 4 and 9.

Changing the Way We Think

An important reason why we often fail to understand our muscle pain is that we commonly start far away from the cause-and-effect logic of the body and the muscular system—which is not surprising, since the necessary information has not been available to us. Typically, all we have ready access to is a lot of diagnostic terms. There are almost too many to chose from: thoracic outlet syndrome, carpal tunnel syndrome, tendinitis, runner's knee, tennis elbow, and many, many more. Naturally, we want to be aware of these so that we can decide if they fit our own situation. However, such conditions do not appear out of nowhere. As you learn how your muscles function and how the different parts of the musculoskeletal system work together, you will understand how pain can develop based on the logic of this system. Furthermore, you will be able to remove, one by one, many of the factors that are causing your pain.

But first, changing the way you think is the first step toward resolving your muscle pain.

Six Myths about Muscle Pain

Even though the logic of cause and effect may be obvious in theory, when you start applying it to your own situation, many habitual thought patterns interfere. The following six powerful myths prevent many of us from successfully relieving our muscle pain:

1. My muscle pain is so complicated that I cannot possibly understand it. Everyone's muscular condition is unique and different. However, painful muscles, wherever located and for whatever reasons, usually have similar traits. If you look at the basics of how the muscles react to changes—for example, changes in posture and activity levels—problems become understandable. Becoming familiar with the general principles of how muscles operate and how they react can give you a new understanding of your own specific problem.

2. Muscle pain is just something I have to live with. There is nothing I can do about it.   If your muscles hurt, they are communicating that something is wrong. And they will continue to hurt until you hear what they are telling you and respond by doing something. When you have learned to follow the signals and respond with activities promoting muscle health, you will begin to experience genuine relief from muscle pain.

3. Stretching does not work for me. I tried it, and it only made the pain worse.   Feelings of increased tightness and pain—maybe even spasms—caused by stretching occur for logical reasons. These sensations are due to monitors in the muscle that regulate and adjust tightness in reaction to a stretch and the way we stretch. Learning what these monitors are and how to stretch in cooperation with them will make the stretch work and stimulate pain-relieving changes. When you understand the mechanisms that are activated in the muscle as you stretch, you will not be surprised at the different sensations in and around the muscle during and after stretching.

4. If I rest my painful muscles, they will heal.   It is true that when you experience an acute injury to muscles or tissue, resting is the best and most appropriate response. Most muscle pain, however, has developed over a long time. The damage has become chronic, and in this situation, resting does not have a healing effect.

5. I exercise, work out, and lift weights. Therefore, my muscle pain will go away. Aerobic exercise, such as walking or running, can be the ultimate cure for pained muscles. It brings fresh, healing blood to the painful areas, helping to improve circulation. However, when you lift weights, you strengthen the muscle fibers. If the muscle is ready to be strengthened and if you know that strengthening one muscle necessitates strengthening the other muscles in its group, lifting weights can be an excellent way to heal muscle pain. But strengthening unevenly, without paying attention to how the muscles work together, can actually launch you into an *increased* cycle of pain, rather than take you out of it!

6. Of course my muscles are painful. That's a natural consequence of aging, and there's nothing I can do about it. Recently, as a result of increased studies of exercise activity in elderly people, a rush of data about how aging really affects the body has emerged. These data prove that it is decreased levels of activity, more than degeneration of muscles and tissue, that cause increased muscle aching with age.

Understanding Your Muscle Condition

This book will show you many ways to provide self-massage to bring relief and healing to your muscles and tissue, as well as how to improve the ranges of movement of your joints and how to impact the tension, length, and strength of your muscles. But the most important thing is how to understand your own condition.

At your first appointment, therapists concentrate on attempting to understand your particular condition. While you may want to hurry on to treatment so you can start to relieve your pain as soon as possible, therapists spend time asking questions, moving things around, observing, and thinking. What they observe provides them with a world of information about your individual muscle condition. This information is exactly what you need to avoid muscle pain. Had you had such information at hand yourself, you most likely would not have needed the therapist at all.

Unfortunately, some therapists forget to provide a running commentary as they carry out their examination, leaving patients in the dark about their own body's condition. Others talk, but in an incomprehensible jargon of complicated terms that obscure the logic and importance of what they are saying. Many therapists, however, explain what they are doing while they perform their information-gathering examination. If you listen carefully, you will discover that they are looking to see how your particular situation deviates from established standards of normal, pain-free movement, strength, and health. Even small deviations can cause large amounts of pain, and small corrections can relieve large amounts of pain.

The message of this book is simple: Much of the muscle pain we experience is unnecessary; not only can it be soothed, but it can be healed and prevented. Most of us take our pain for granted. We have been dealing with stiff, aching knees and sore lower backs for so many years. We have given up on our favorite activities because they cause more pain than enjoyment and have reserved our visits to the doctor for more "serious" complaints because we did not think there was anything we could do about it. When we learn to understand and work with the versatility of the muscular system, the thinking patterns that have kept us from restoring our muscular health will be replaced by productive knowledge and pain-relieving skills we can apply every day.

We do not have to live with muscle pain, and healing need not entail painful, expensive, and time-consuming treatment.

Who Is This Book For?

This book has been designed to be used under a variety of conditions: whether you are a patient under a doctor's and/or therapist's care or simply someone who has been coping for years with aches and pains you didn't know you could do something about.

Terms

A time when you are in pain is not the best time to learn a new vocabulary. Therefore, we have decided to use the following descriptive words and phrases instead of medical terms:

• *Key muscles* are the 36 muscles we have chosen to present in this book. There are many more muscles in the body, but these are for the most part primary movers of your joints. The idea is that when you learn how these 36 muscles work, you will be able to use medical books on your own to study other muscles that might be relevant to your condition.

• *Muscle job* describes the motion the muscle is causing at a joint.

- *Bony landmarks* are the important landmarks in the body for finding the muscles and their attachment sites, which is a large part of the method used to treat the muscles in this book. These are names such as "small outer elbow bone" instead of *lateral epicondyle* and "tip of the shoulder" instead of *acromion process.* You will get comfortable with these terms as you use the book, since they are used consistently throughout.

- A muscle attaches to the bone in two places. We will use *beginning tendon* to describe the attachment closest to the center of the body, where the tendon attaches to a relatively stable bone. This replaces the medical term *origin. Ending tendon* will be used to describe an attachment usually farther away from the center of the body, where the tendon attaches to a more mobile bone. This replaces the medical term *insertion.*

- *Primary mover* (which replaces the medical term *agonist*) describes the muscle that is mainly responsible for a movement, for example, bending the trunk forward. The *opposing muscle* (which replaces the medical term *antagonist*) is the muscle that does the exact opposite of the primary mover, and *assisting muscles* (which replaces the medical term *synergists*) help the primary mover.

- *Abuse* describes any kind of overuse, misuse, or injury to a muscle.

CHAPTER 2

Rethinking Muscle Pain

It is still amazing to me how I recovered from the many age-old aches and pains that used to plague my body. For a long time, I tried my best to put these pains out of my mind, so I never expected—or planned—to rid myself of any of them.

The turnaround started with an injury to my wrist and elbow. The recovery from this painful condition was long, frustrating, and confusing. No one could explain why the injury did not heal despite the many different treatments I was receiving. I spent six months unable to work full-time at my computer. The exercises I had been given seemed to aggravate my pain and swelling, so I stopped doing them out of fear. I was ready to give up when I finally met a therapist who told me that the only way to recover was to give the muscle fibers sufficient blood flow over time, which would allow them to heal. Persistent massaging of my arm, stretching, and finally strengthening brought me back to full-time work in just a few weeks.

This experience made me wonder: What exactly is muscle pain, since it could so easily go away after being a problem for so long? I learned that all muscles basically function and heal the same way. This encouraged me to start treating and stretching other areas of my body where I had muscular pain, such as my aching lower back, my tense shoulders, a hip that periodically ached during winter nights, and the knee that hurt when walking up the steps in my backyard.

I started to carefully and systematically apply the exact same steps to these areas as I had to my arm injury. I massaged, stretched, and persisted even if there was pain. The key was to accept a little worsening at the beginning of the healing process. What seemed to be a miracle happened. Step by step, muscle by muscle, joint by joint, the different chronic pains went away, some surprisingly swiftly and others more slowly.

I cannot, even if I try to, recall the feeling of my aching hip as I turned around in bed; even the pain in my lower back that used to make me dread getting out of bed is a faded memory.

—Elisabeth

What You Can Do to Help Heal Your Muscles

Most of us are acutely aware that physical and emotional stress immediately impacts our neck and back muscles, as well as those in our legs and arms. We can't seem to stop our muscles from tensing up and developing painful knots, and so we conclude that we also cannot relieve them of tension and pain. However, just as stress and tension coming from within have great consequences for how our muscles behave, anything that is imposed on the body from the outside also has a large influence. Take, for example, your body's reaction to cold weather. The muscles tighten up, often leaving your body stiff and aching. On the other hand, think of how soft and relaxed the muscles feel after a hot bath. Recall how sitting for long hours in one position causes the muscles to ache, and then how a good back rub can relieve a lot of muscle tension.

When the sensation and condition of our muscles change, this is due to physiological changes within the circulatory and nervous systems in our body. These systems are very sensitive and are designed to respond instantly to any changes imposed on the body, internal or external. Since they consist of blood vessels and nerves, which are everywhere in the body, we can get to them and have an impact on them by working from the outside, as well as by working with processes within the body.

We often believe that the magic of physical therapy and massage is the only thing that can make us feel good again. A skilled therapist makes joints that were restricted move more easily, releases the pain in muscles that were tense and sore, and allows us to breathe more easily. The magic is simply that the muscles and tissues respond to manual treatment, sometimes with immediate pain relief and enhanced well-being.

You, too, can learn to take advantage of this opportunity to reduce pain and improve your muscles' condition. You will be surprised at how much you can accomplish with your own hands and your own treatment strategy.

What Is Muscle Pain?

Consider the following examples:

Example A: If you run up a hill too fast or carry a load that is too heavy, you will soon experience discomfort or burning pain in your muscles. When you stop the activity, the pain soon goes away.

But most of our muscle pain does not go away when we stop our activities, nor does it arise from suddenly overworking the muscles. It is closer to the next example.

Example B: If you obstruct the flow of blood to your hand and forearm muscles—for example, by tying a rope tightly around your upper arm—and then perform some activity with that hand, you will experience a painful sensation in your arm within minutes. If you continue the activity, this pain can soon reach intolerable levels. When you stop the activity, you will find that the pain does not go away by itself. It lingers on, and the pain does not go away until you remove the rope and move your arm.

There is an important difference between these two examples. In Example A—sudden hard activity—the circulation cannot keep up with the demand of the muscle fibers for blood flow. The starving fibers scream for oxygen and nutrients, and the result is pain. But when you stop running or lifting, the muscle fibers recover quickly as blood rushes freely back into your muscles. Within minutes you are pain-free.

In Example B, the circulation is again insufficient. The muscles use up the available oxygen and nutrients and do not receive enough replacements. The pain signals that the muscle fibers need fresh blood. In this case, however, stopping the activity will not take the pain away. This is due to the tightness in the upper arm where the rope is still so tight around the arm that the blood is prevented from flowing back in.

What happens in both examples forms the basis for the most common experiences of muscle pain. Any form of reduced blood flow to your muscle fibers has the potential to cause quite a lot of discomfort and pain. Likewise, removing obstructions that reduce blood flow can relieve large amounts of pain.

The Waste Products

To find the source of the pain in your muscles, you must look to the waste products—wastes left over from muscle work when nutrients from the blood are used up. Waste products are continuously produced and washed out by blood circulation as we move or exercise. In Example A above, the suddenly hardworking muscle fibers produced waste products faster than blood circulation could provide new nutrients. In Example B, the obstruction limited blood supply to the arm, and the waste products being produced were not washed out effectively. The net result in both cases was lack of oxygen and waste product overflow—and pain.

Your body constantly attempts to maintain a balance (*homeostasis*) among the different substances in the body. It alerts your brain when a significant imbalance exists. The waste products contain chemical substances, which must be present in the body in balanced amounts. With proper balance, there is no pain. When blood flow is reduced, however, the waste products are not washed away and the level of chemicals increases beyond the acceptable level for your body. The result is familiar: We are in pain. The aching, soreness, and sensitivity that we know so well are the result.

You can now imagine what happens when the circulation is *cut off*, as in Example B: Large amounts of waste products containing these chemicals are produced. The waste remains in the tissue around the nerve endings (tiny branches of the nerve where it ends in the tissue), and you experience an intolerable burning pain when the nerve endings start firing off messages to the brain. These nerve endings are particularly sensitive to such chemicals. Assuming the blood starts rushing through your muscles and tissue again, the pain can sometimes disappear in as little as 10 to 20 seconds!

Quick Relief

When your muscles hurt:

- Gently massage the painful area
- Slowly stretch the muscles and tissue
- Use hot and cold packs alternately to increase the circulation of blood (See Chapter 5)
- Repeat these steps frequently

Thus, muscle pain is usually not a sign that there is something violent or destructive going on in our muscles. Rather, pain is a result of the messages about substance imbalance being conveyed between the nerves and the brain. This definition may sound too simplistic for something that really hurts, yet this is the basic mechanism for the sensation of muscle pain.

When you understand the cycle of nutrients and oxygen in your blood circulating in the muscles, you can begin to understand why and how you can enhance the well-being and health of your muscles and greatly contribute to healing. It is helpful to study how this happens in the body.

The Circulation of Blood

Most of us know that it is important to drink a lot of water and eat healthy foods. Of course we are aware that the things we eat and drink pass through the digestive system, but we often forget that the process that actually keeps us alive is the one by which food is absorbed into the bloodstream and transported around the body by the blood. This blood is also circulated through all the organs and tissue in the body, including our muscles.

An understanding of this cycle reveals valuable tools available to us for relieving pain and keeping the muscles healthy. To clarify this, we can divide blood circulation into three parts: blood going to the muscles, blood going through the muscles, and blood going from the muscles. Anything that occurs along this three-stage path immediately affects the health of the muscle.

Blood Going to the Muscles

The blood flowing to the muscles is newly oxygenated, fresh from the heart, and contains everything the muscles need to be healthy and thrive as long as we make sure our blood gets the right nutrients through our diet.

We hear a lot about nutrition and a healthy diet, but there is yet another factor to consider that does not get as much press: We must also ensure that the blood actually reaches the muscles. If the vessels that transport blood from the heart encounter obstructions along any point on their route, this will affect the blood supply to the muscles.

Our daily activities, postural habits, tension, stress, and use and abuse of our muscles can cause subtle changes to the tissues in the body. Physical and massage therapists report that by palpating muscles and tissue, they find these changes in the form of, for example, excess tissue (scar tissue), small areas of swelling (edema), and chronically contracted muscle fibers. Although we are unaware of such changes, they can form obstructions that cause the blood vessels and nerves to become squeezed and compressed, allowing less blood to reach the muscles and nerves.

Blood Going through the Muscles

Let us assume the blood has been successfully transported to the muscle. What happens next? The long, thick-walled blood vessels carrying blood away from the heart to the body (the arteries) only transport the blood. The tissue, organs, and muscles do not actually receive the blood supply until it enters the tiny blood vessels inside the muscles, the capillaries. The capillaries are quite abundant in muscle tissue. They are small, thin-walled, permeable blood vessels that allow the nutrients carried in the blood to pass through their walls. This is where the ultimate function of the entire cardiovascular system is performed: the supplying of nutrients and the removal of waste products.

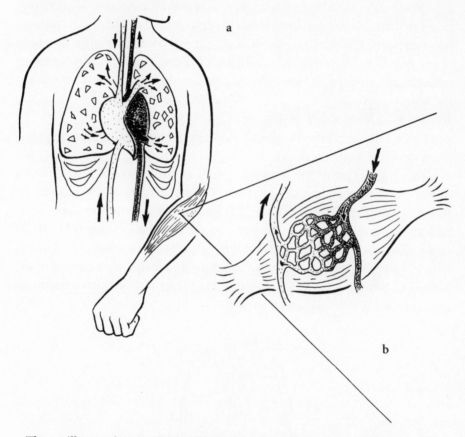

The capillary exchange: (a) blood flow to (dark) and from (white) all the tissue, muscles, and organs in the body; (b) blood flow through a muscle.

Inside the muscles—whether they are sore, weak, strong, or healthy—is where the vitamins, minerals, and even the water we take in are utilized, as well as where the alcohol and coffee we consume pass through (after the stomach, intestines, and liver have done their job). Here is also where the waste products are washed out and replaced with nutrients. Much depends on this exchange, and it is crucial that it occur with few obstructions.

Healthy muscles are continually replenished with fresh nutrients and oxygen and cleaned of wastes and are therefore better able to withstand stress and resist eventual damage. On the other hand, if there are obstructions to the blood flow, the exchange can be slowed, or worse, prevented from happening at all. For example, muscle contraction itself produces large compressional forces within the muscle and the tissue. This in turn can press on the blood vessels and prevent blood flow. A sustained contraction can actually stop the blood flow completely. After such a contraction, however, during relaxation, the flow resumes at an even higher rate than usual. Effective absorption and exchange of nutrients in the muscles are as essential as supplying the required nutrition to the body in the first place.

Blood Going from the Muscles

After blood transportation and nutrient delivery, one vital process remains: the removal of waste products.

The contraction of the muscles is itself an important part of cleaning out the waste products they produce. We are used to the idea that the pumping of the heart drives the whole circulatory system. But the heart is basically responsible mainly for the first part of the job, pumping fresh, clean blood out to the tissues. We rely greatly on our muscles and the lymph system for the second part. The muscles are the main drivers in the process of pumping the old blood back to get cleaned, through a pumping system called the *skeletal muscle pump.*

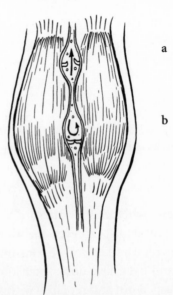

The skeletal muscle pump: (a) an open valve; (b) a closed valve.

When we exercise, this pump works at full speed. It is so efficient because of the valves inside the veins, which allow the old blood to flow only in one direction, back to the heart. The more we exercise, the more blood containing waste products we send out of the tissue, and the more room is created for nutritious new blood to enter. The better the condition our muscles are in, the more efficient this process is. We therefore depend on healthy muscles to keep our muscles healthy.

Each part of the circulation, each influencing the effectiveness of the others, contains helpful hints for you regarding how you can relieve your muscles of pain. Utilizing these hints, the improvement in your muscle condition can be remarkable!

Thoughts and Feelings

Still, the many different sensations in your muscles throughout the course of your daily activities, while moving, sitting still, doing stretches, or lying down, can be hard to decipher. You might not be sure whether the pain is telling you to be more careful, to stop what you are doing, or, conversely, to increase your activity. When you start realizing how predictably it appears and goes away, you are less likely to worry as much about it. Taking away the fear of muscle pain makes it much easier to relieve.

How effectively you are able to work toward relieving pain in your muscles greatly depends on your thoughts and feelings. Exercise soreness, for example, is no joke: stretching, walking up stairs, or simply getting through the day moving normally can be extremely painful. Yet most people tolerate it with good spirits. Other muscular pains may be less intense but are experienced as worse, due to our fears about the possible unknown causes.

Instincts

A recent newspaper article announced: "If you have back pain, do not sit still—MOVE it!" Movement reduces pain and promotes healing. Even if your instincts tell you not to move when it hurts, your success at relieving muscle pain greatly depends on how much you generate motion in and around your aching muscles. It can seem counterintuitive that your instinct would cause you to protect and keep the muscles still when this is exactly the opposite of what leads to healing. But your instincts are not fooling you, they are perfectly sound. Their role is to make sure you are alerted to a situation that requires your attention and care. You are being reminded to produce healing conditions. However, you don't always respond by doing the right thing for the situation. Learning to distinguish between the different kinds of pain will guide you to do the things that lead to healing and relief.

Different Kinds of Pain

The kind of pain you have determines what you should do about it.

Acute pain is the kind you feel when you stub your toe, suffer a burn, or experience a wound to your flesh. It is clear that an injury is occurring, or the circumstances are such that they will lead to immediate injury if nothing is done. Instinctively, you do the right thing without giving it a second thought, namely, staying still and caring for the wound as it heals.

Such acute pain decreases over time, during which the main process is the healing of the injury. Acute pain, therefore, is a warning to stay immobile so the wound can best heal.

Most muscle pain is not acute pain, unless the pain is related to a recent injury. Most often, our muscle pain stems from a process that has developed over time and become *chronic*. The buildup is so slow in and around the muscle that the condition may have been with you for a long time before you noticed the pain. In a situation of chronic muscle pain, the healing phase is over. The period of time during which the injury or wound healed has passed. Actual healing is not going on any longer.

The pain does not go away with time unless some action is taken. This is exactly what most people do not realize. We tend to think that by resting and being careful, which our instincts tell us to do, the pain will eventually disappear. The pain *will* go away, but only if we do what it takes to heal it.

Any pain that persists for more than six weeks is considered chronic. When the pain persists even after the cause of the pain is known and has been treated, the pain has settled in the body. Although some periods may be less pain-filled than others, overall the pain remains very much the same. However, more than other chronic pains, chronic muscle pain can be worked with and changed for the better. After removing the factors that maintain the chronic state, even pain that has been with us for many years can be successfully cured.

Chronic muscle pain does no real harm. It is not a symptom of a threatening change or a warning to stay immobile, and is not a pain state that is asking for rest. In fact, since muscle pain is very often the result of long-term restriction of blood flow to the muscle, remaining immobile has no beneficial effect; on the contrary, it can make the pain worse. Chronic muscle pain will not diminish, heal, and go away unless you move the muscle.

Chronic waste overload causes chronic pain. The nerve endings are chronically irritated. As a result of this constant stimulation, they tend to actually increase in sensitivity, eventually becoming hyperirritable. A fitting analogy is the kind of hyperirritable person for whom an inconse-quential remark provokes a disproportionately huge and inappropriate reaction. Even a tiny stimulation sends a flood of pain messages to the brain, even though there has been no increase in the cause of the pain. The problem now lies in the signaling process. There is no real cause of pain any longer. The pain is more like a false alarm.

Although such pain can be very uncomfortable, it does not pose an immediate or significant threat, whether limited to a small area or extend-ing across whole muscle groups. Most who suffer from such chronic pain are not aware of this process. Therefore, it is not uncommon to develop a fear of moving to avoid aggravating the pain.

How can you determine whether a particular pain feeling stems from acute or chronic pain? If you experience sharp, strong, and unfamiliar pain, your first step should be to check with a doctor to rule out every pos-sible source of pain that might be caused by illness, broken bones, rheuma-tism, or other conditions. As you grow more experienced with the features of muscle pain, you will more readily be able to tell the difference yourself.

The Pain Cycle

It can be truly hard to escape from chronic muscle pain unless you have an understanding of how it maintains itself in the body. You may have tried working out, stretching, and many other techniques to rid yourself of pain, without achieving the results you expected. If you did not succeed, it was very likely due to the way chronic pain establishes a cycle that perpetually goes around and around. The cycle must be broken in order for you to effectively rid yourself of pain.

First, let us look, very roughly, at how this cycle becomes established: Each pain message sent from the nerve endings to the brain calls for an action. When the nervous system receives the message, it tells the muscles, "Do something!" The muscles respond by contracting—even if just on a microscopic level (microspasms). Contraction produces waste products, which send increased pain messages to the brain. This, in turn, causes the brain to order more microcontraction. The very message about pain has become the cause of even more pain in the muscle. This cycle of pain can continue in a self-sustained and chronic spiral in which the muscles slowly become ever more tense and painful.

For some, the pain cycle is limited to the shoulder area. For some, it may only exist in the elbow area. For others, the hip, knee, and foot may also be involved. The chronic pain cycle can include many muscle groups, making you feel as if you hurt all over, all the time. The importance of breaking this cycle and relieving muscle pain becomes clear when you understand that the cycle can stay constant but can also gradually intensify, causing affected muscles to become tighter.

When you know how this cycle is established, step by step, muscle fiber by muscle fiber, you will know to break it by eliminating the factors that built it, step by step. You can start wherever there is soreness, tightness, lack of flexibility, and lack of strength. These conditions cause obstructions to the flow of blood and keep your muscles locked in the pain cycle. Then you can deliberately start to remove the pain-creating factors, one after the other, at a pace suited to your condition. When you get to know your body, you will find the tempo that fits your condition. You can turn the pain cycle around. You do not have to be paralyzed by your muscle pain.

Turn a Bad Day into a Learning Tool

A bad day, when the aching is especially strong, is—contrary to what you might feel—the best day to start caring for your hurting muscles. This does not mean that it's the best time to start drastic work on tissue and muscles, because on such days your system most likely is overloaded and won't be able to carry away the wastes effectively. But a bad day does offer a golden opportunity for gathering information. At no other time does your body reveal such a wealth of detailed information about the pattern of the dams, or blocks, in your circulation. (If you do not experience really bad days, early mornings are also good for this purpose. For most of us, it is when we awaken in the morning and start to move that the old familiar stiff and achy places make themselves known.) Your aches disclose the exact locations of your most vulnerable and hurt muscles and which motions (muscle jobs) are involved in your pain. This is the time to take notes.

Ask yourself the following questions:

When Does It Hurt?   On days like today? More important, after days like yesterday?

Why Does It Hurt?   What did you do before you experienced the pain? Could this be the cause? Did you lift something heavy, sit on a plane for a long time, experience a very stressful time, sleep in a certain position, type on a keyboard, use a power drill, or sew on a sewing machine?

Where Does It Hurt?   Note the exact location. Is it close to a bone, or in the soft areas of the muscle?

How Does It Hurt?   Note the quality of the pain. Is it sharp, dull, or deep, aching pain?

After you have gathered all the information you can get from your aching joints and muscles—make sure you do not miss this opportunity—you will now posses a wealth of knowledge that will put you in charge of your muscle pain. Step by step, you will be able to remove the obstructions that drive your pain cycle, whether it is tiny or more expansive.

Remember: Movement is essential, even when muscles are painful. Movement increases blood flow, providing an emergency supply of nutrients and oxygen to the muscle fibers and giving them a chance to heal. And when muscles are tight and tension-filled, movement contributes to restoring normal length and tension to tightened muscle fibers, which is necessary for healing.

By treating pain as a guide to oxygen-starved areas, you are providing yourself with a new and surprising tool to get rid of it. You cannot expect to rid yourself of all your chronic muscle pain in 10 to 20 seconds. But be assured that you *can* relieve such pain. Pain that has existed for a shorter time can respond almost immediately to treatment. Older pains may take awhile to disappear.

Experiencing this process at work, and changing your thinking to embrace the truth that you can relieve the pain in your muscles through movement, builds the courage and optimism to do it more often. Soon, working with and through muscle pain becomes a habit.

Breaking the Cycle

Think positively—you *can* relieve your pain!

Become aware of your muscle's health by:

- Locating and being mindful of tightness in your muscles.
- Locating and paying attention to sore and tender areas.
- Testing your joint's range of motion.
- Checking your muscles for symptoms of weakness.

Routinely, during your daily activities:

- Stimulate the circulation in every way possible to help wash out waste products.
- Stretch whenever your muscles feel tight, relieving them as tightness appears.
- Reverse your habitual movement patterns by stretching the other side.
- Strengthen weak muscles so that they never deteriorate into the lose–lose scenario of the pain cycle.

CHAPTER 3

What Are Muscles, Tendons, and Ligaments?

"Is there anyone in this town who can tell me anything about tendons?" I cried out in despair. The doctor had said: "You have carpal tunnel syndrome. Let me explain: The finger flexor muscles run over the carpal bones and under the transverse ligament, a tough membrane that holds the bones together. We call this the carpal tunnel. When the connective tissue and sheath of these tendons start to swell, the median nerve becomes compressed. We can relieve the pain in your wrist by releasing the nerve from its entrapment during surgery." I had nodded. I felt the doctor had done a good job explaining, and what he said had sounded as if it should be so obvious. I felt that I should have known the terms he used and was too embarrassed to admit I did not even know what a tendon was.

I looked at my wrist. My mind went blank when I tried to imagine what was under the skin.

—Rebecca

What's Under Your Skin?

Trying to picture how the pieces fit and work together under the skin can be very confusing. It is much like looking under the hood of a car for the first time. However, knowing the different parts, their uses, and how they interact helps you to maintain and heal your muscles. Most of us do not really know what these critically fundamental parts of our bodies look like and how they work together under the skin. The purpose of this chapter is to help you imagine some of the structures and processes of your muscles, tendons, and connective tissue so you can know in more detail what it is you treat.

The Muscles

What Is a Muscle?

Generally speaking, a muscle is a sac containing many bundles of muscle fibers. Each bundle resides in its own sac of tissue, and each narrow muscle fiber is likewise in a sac.

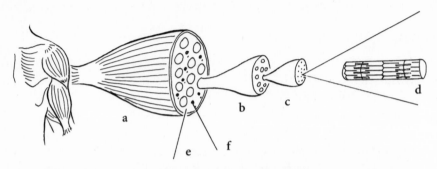

Inside a muscle: (a) a muscle sac; (b) a bundle of fibers; (c) a single fiber; (d) contraction threads; (e) a nerve; (f) a blood vessel.

Still, a muscle appears as a whole entity because the outermost sac holds its content firmly together and ties it to the bone. The number of the extremely thin, long fibers inside a muscle varies, but it is always a large quantity. For example, an average front thigh muscle can contain more than a million individual fibers!

The muscle is divided into three parts: the muscle belly, which is the large soft part containing the bundles of fibers, and the two attachment sites, which are the ends of the muscle tissue, the tendons, that attach to the bone. Both ends of the muscle must be attached, so a muscle usually has at least two tendons.

You can feel the muscle bellies by touching, rubbing, or pressing on the soft parts of your arms, legs, neck, or shoulders. They are soft when relaxed but harden when they contract.

Find a Muscle and Feel It Move

Find the muscle that bends the foot up toward the shinbone (tibialis anterior).

- Sit with your knees bent. Place your fingers in the middle of the shinbone about two inches under the end of the kneecap. Move your fingers an inch toward the outer side of the leg.

- Hold here while you bend your foot up (dorsiflexion), and feel the muscle harden under your fingers as it contracts.

Inside the muscles is a rich, elaborate network of blood vessels and nerves, able to stretch along with the muscle. These penetrate every tiny part of a muscle. The large amount of blood vessels creates the muscles' red color.

Muscle Fibers

Contraction, muscle damage, and strength-building all happen inside each single muscle fiber. The fiber is long and cylindrical in shape, red or light pink in color, and often extends along the whole muscle length. In some muscles, the fibers can be as long as 20 centimeters.

The Mechanisms of Muscle Contraction

Muscle contraction is the function of "motors" that lie inside the fiber. One single motor is only a tiny section (sarcomere) of the long fiber, which consists of many, many such sections extending along its length.

You can roughly visualize how contraction happens within a section of a muscle fiber if you hold your hands up, palms facing you and pointing the fingertips toward each other. Spread your fingers slightly and let them slide in between each other until the fingertips are stopped at the base of them. Now, let them slide back out until the fingertips no longer touch. These two positions of your fingers approximately simulate full contraction and full stretch within a motor. Your fingers represent a set of parallel contraction threads (actin and myosinfilaments) that slide closer when the muscle contracts. When you imagine a long row of these tiny motors working, you can understand how refined the contraction of a muscle is.

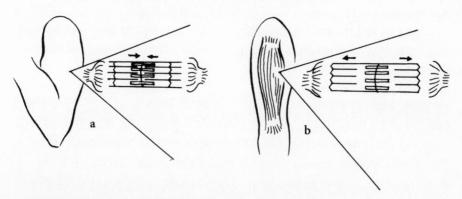

Contracted and stretched muscle fiber: (a) contracted fiber; (b) stretched fiber.

The motors are turned on and off by messages transmitted through the nerve that supplies the fiber. A message from the central nervous system, starting in the brain at the top of the spinal cord, travels down the nerve to the muscle fiber. Here, it is transformed into a local chemical process that in turn causes the threads to start sliding. The whole process takes only a fraction of a second to complete, generating force and movement in an instant.

NERVES

A nerve is a path between the central nervous system and the tissue of your muscles. The nerve needs plenty of oxygen to operate the muscles' motors properly. Sustained pressure on a nerve from any kind of obstruction in the body can cause lack of oxygen (ischemia), which can cause a nerve to fire too often, causing too tight, too tense (hypertonic) muscles, or fire too slowly and too seldom, causing flaccid muscles. Light tingling, slight numbness, or too much contraction in the muscles can be symptoms that the nerve is not getting enough oxygen.

Muscle Damage and Fiber Tear—Part of Nature's Design

When muscle fibers contract, the fibers are often roughed up in many different ways. We call this "muscle damage" or "fiber tearing." This is not real damage, but microscopic tearing that is part of a natural process, and is designed to occur. Thus, muscle fiber tearing is not an injury in itself. Fiber rupture and repair happen all the time as we move and exercise.

Strength

The building of strength in a muscle means that there has been fiber tearing, that the tiny tears have been repaired, and that new cells have replaced damaged ones. However, the repair must be complete. If the repair process is not efficient, real injury is close at hand. Muscle fiber repair demands a large supply of blood.

Healing Muscle Fibers

Regular everyday actions constantly move the fibers and stimulate the circulation inside them, bringing healing and nutritious blood to the muscle. This is why people often say that muscles repair themselves. If, however, there are obstructions in the tissue, the blood flow might be inhibited and your muscles may not heal as well. You can help the healing process significantly by increasing the blood flow.

Quick Relief for a Tight Muscle

- Carefully rub the muscle belly, which brings oxygen to the fibers.
- Carefully and thoroughly rub the bones close to the sore muscle, which brings oxygen to the tendon that attaches to the bones.
- Slowly stretch the muscle while you breathe deeply, which most effectively brings oxygen to each part of the muscle.

All of the above helps increase blood flow.

Tension and Length Regulation

A monitoring system inside the fibers detects changes in length and tension, telling the central nervous system to adjust when needed. This system (see pages 72–73) is so central that you cannot massage or stretch your muscles without activating it. In fact, you activate it any time you move. The system works to sustain your posture and allow movement. This happens through a combination of maintaining the fibers at the same length (you feel this as a pulling back when you stretch), which is necessary to sustain posture, and adapting to the changes in length, which is necessary for movement. Therapists work with these mechanisms that so powerfully control our muscles.

THE STRETCH REFLEX

When you stretch a muscle you will feel the *stretch reflex*, a temporary pullback inside the fibers before they release. The monitoring system is at work. The more speed you stretch with, the harder the pullback is.

The Latin Names of the Muscles

Do you need to bother with these? Getting to know them can be well worth the effort, even if it seems confusing at first. They become easier to remember when you see that they all have a meaning that helps you remember them. The names can refer to:

- The size of the muscle, using terms such as *maximus* (large), *minimus* (small), or *longus* (long). For example, gluteus maximus literally means "large buttocks."

- The location of the muscle, using terms like *anterior* (front) or *posterior* (back). For example, tibialis anterior literally means "close to tibia in front."
- The shape of the muscle, like the trapezius, meaning a shape that has four sides (trapezoid).

Tendons

What Is a Tendon?

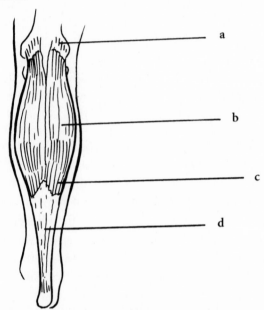

A tendon: (a) tendon; (b) muscle belly; (c) junction between
muscle and tendon fibers; (d) tendon

All the tissue that wraps each individual muscle fiber comes together where the muscle's sac ends. This is the tendon, a sheath of tissue that attaches the muscle to the bone. The word tendon stems from the Latin word *tendere*, which means "to stretch."

Tendinitis, inflammation of the tendon fibers, can develop when the tendon is under too much stress while receiving too little nutrition from blood circulation. Learning about how tendons work can help you treat and prevent this.

You can see how tendons are attached to bones when you take the meat (the muscle) off the bone of a chicken, but how can you tell a tendon from a muscle in your own body? As a rule of thumb, when you move your fingers away from the soft part—the muscle belly—and closer to the bone, you are likely to find this muscle's tendon because this is where it attaches.

Several tendons are easy to find and feel. You can feel and see the finger tendons on the back of your hand if you make a fist. The hard ropes that lie just under the skin are the tendons from the finger muscles, whose bellies go up the forearm to the elbow. The finger tendons are surrounded by a sheath filled with fluid that permits them to move without friction and without being irritated by surrounding parts like bones, ligaments, and other muscles. Those sheaths are what you see on the back of the hand. If you sit with your knees bent, you can feel the thick tendon ropes that attach the large hamstring muscles to the back of the knee.

Find a Tendon and Feel It Move

Find the Achilles tendon, the tendon of the calf muscles.

- Sit with your knee bent. Place your fingers on the back of your ankle (1.5 inches above the heel bone) where you feel a hard surface.
- Lift your heel and feel this tendon tighten under your fingers.
- Follow the tendon in both directions, down the ankle to the heel bone, where it attaches, and up the lower leg until it widens out and becomes the calf muscle.

You can find other tendons by looking at the illustrations in Chapter 9, which show every tendon attachment for each key muscle.

BONE PAIN OR MUSCLE PAIN?

The tendons attach to the bone in such a way that they almost merge with the bone. Sometimes tendons even grow into the bone. Therefore, pain from an injured tendon very often feels as if originates in the bone.

When you treat sore tendon attachments you may be surprised at how many of the aching bone pains, even deep, aching pain in hips, shoulders and knees, go away and do not return.

Tendons come in many shapes and sizes: long, thin, short, flat sheets, round, big, and small. Large, strong muscles usually have short, flat tendons, whereas muscles that perform delicate movements have long, thin tendons. Sometimes tendons feel like thick ropes or stringy threads; at times they feel hard as bone, and sometimes as if made of a squishy gel.

Tendon Fibers

The tendon is a part of the muscle, yet very different from it. Its fibers are white and glistening. Even though it is not red like the muscle fibers, there are small blood vessels, nerves, and lymphatic vessels in between the fibers of most tendons. These extend into the deeper portion of the tendon.

Tendons are strong and tough, like steel, thanks to the crisscross pattern of the fibers, and can be pulled in many directions. If they are pulled slowly and carefully, they can withstand a great load (500–1,000 kg). But if they are jerked or loaded very rapidly, they can still rupture. Surgeons who have operated on them understand their phenomenal strength. After cutting a tendon, they are often unable to hold the muscle stretched out with their hands because the muscle contracts so powerfully. You can imagine the constant pressure tendons are under, pulled between the contracting muscle fibers and the hard bone.

Quick Relief for Sore Hips

A common sore spot in the hip is on the outside of the thigh, right where the body bends when you sit. This is the top of the thigh bone (greater trochanter); (to find it, see Chapter 9). Major muscles that move the hip attach on this bone.

- With your thumbs, press in and make small circles on and closely around this bone. Rub, press, and massage, and pay attention to tender areas. (They often need extra work.)
- Rhythmically press in and let go on the sides, under, and above this bone. This helps pump blood through the area.
- End with a slow hip stretch (see Chapter 12).

Tendon injuries do not happen for no reason. Tendons, like muscles, adapt to levels of usage. With little usage, they become weaker. When we suddenly need the tendon's strength in recreation or on the job, the strength may not be there and the load, whether repetitive or sudden, can lead to injury.

Healing Tendon Fibers

Tendons are in a different position than the muscle fibers when it comes to healing. They do not seem to heal by themselves. Therefore, tendinitis can stick around for decades. Today, however, therapists find that tendons heal at faster rates when treated with plenty of motion and blood flow stimulation. The areas close around the tendon are very good places to massage to provide extra blood flow. Exercise and stretching make tendons stronger and more resistant to injuries.

Quick Relief for Elbow Pain

- Bend your elbow and with your other hand locate the bony bumps of your elbow (see Chapter 9).
- With your thumb, rub in small circles on and below these bones, about an inch or two down on the forearm. (The major muscles that move the wrist and fingers attach to these bones.)
- Rub across the forearm right below the elbow, pressing deeply to stir the circulation. Note ropy, sore areas. (They need extra work.)
- End with a slow stretch (wrist and finger stretches in Chapter 12).

Quick Relief for Sore Knees

- With both your thumbs working together, find the bony bumps on and closely positioned around the knee joint (see Chapter 9). (These bumps are where the major muscles that move the knee attach.)
- Press in and move your thumbs in small circles on and closely around every bone you can feel. Rub, press, and massage each one—and work extra on tender spots.
- End with a slow stretch of the thigh and leg muscles (see Chapter 12).

Connective Tissue

Tendons connect a muscle to a bone. Ligaments connect a bone to another bone. Both are connective tissue. The tissue that wraps, packs, connects, and holds each muscle fiber and connects one organ to another (fascia) is another kind. Yet another type, areolar tissue, a network of watery, silky thin tissue, forms a whole unbroken membrane of connective tissue running under the skin and in between every tiny individual part of the body. It extends from the deepest cavities of the organs to the superficial layer under the skin.

We are not much aware of the connective tissue, yet it is where many obstructions to the blood flow to our muscles and nerves develop. Scar tissue and adhesions are invisible villains in our connective tissue system that we can learn to discover, treat, and heal.

Connective tissue supports and holds together the parts of the body no matter what happens. If an injury occurs, it must still give support to the joints and muscles. It adapts by building extra tissue around the injury, thickening, tightening, expanding, and bracing in areas where this is needed. When a cut, tear, or wound happens in its fibers, it glues the wound back together by forming scar tissue. It has the ability to adapt to changes in the body. It expands when the muscles increase in girth and shrinks when the muscles diminish in width or length. It also lengthens, shortens, stretches, and changes with the many demands of our different movement patterns and postural positions. In addition, it also contains large amounts of lymphatic vessels and blood vessels that wash out toxins in the body. Because connective tissue is everywhere and creates the environment that muscles, organs, vessels, and nerves live in, its health is of vital importance to the health of the muscles. When it is healthy, it allows free movement and can be likened to layers upon layers of fine silk gliding, rolling, and moving over each other. This allows organs, muscles, bones, nerves, and blood vessels to glide freely in rhythm with the body's internal movement without resistance, friction, or irritation.

SCAR TISSUE

Scar tissue is more than a scar on the outside of the body. It can be found anywhere inside your body where there has been tissue repair. It consists of new collagen fibers that are produced whenever the connective tissue is harmed, hit, torn, or denied a healthy blood supply for a long period of time. Sometimes it is produced in excess. It is a support tissue for weak areas and becomes scars (thickened, hardened, folded, or lumpy tissue).

You can find and feel it if you palpate your tissue in an area of injury.

You can break down and heal scar tissue over time through massage, heat, and slow, careful stretching.

ADHESIONS

Adhesions are hardened, tight, connective tissue like the scar tissue, but instead of new tissue it is old tissue fibers that have glued to each other. These respond well to the same treatment as scar tissue. The glue has the ability to dissolve, so your adhesions disappear.

When connective tissue is tight, injured, and scarred, it can restrict movement and in many ways impede blood circulation. The muscles and organs then can be said to have a condition similar to what happens when you wear clothes that are too tight. Motion becomes uncomfortable and strained. Normal fascia, although not as strong as tendons and ligaments, has great tensile strength and thus can exert considerable pressure on the body when it tightens.

Because the connective tissue is so changeable, there are many ways you can bring it back to health.

HEALING CONNECTIVE TISSUE

Slow, careful stretching (not overstretching) helps the new and weak collagen fibers strengthen. It also aligns fibers that have become misaligned. This contributes to their health.

Massage helps to circulate fluids to dried-out tissue.

Contraction, stretching, and movement also encourage the pumping of fluids through tissue, helping to carry the wastes away.

The Wake-Up Call

For a variety of reasons, our muscles sometimes do not seem to fully stop contracting. They often keep pulling tighter even after the movement has ended, and the muscles and tissue become sore and painful. Instead of functioning up to their normal potential, some fibers in our muscles get caught in the pain cycle. Much research has been conducted to try to understand this problem, which leads to so much pain for many people, but few certain answers are available.

Therapists have found that many patients experience altered muscular patterns. Their muscles either have increased tone (hypertone) or are weakened, allowing the assisting muscles in their group to take over their job. Both hypertonic and weakened muscles can become troublemakers in the body because problems in one muscle transfer to other muscles (see Chapter 4). Such altered muscle patterns can lead to a lot of pain. Many adults have troublemaker muscles from old injuries or long-term overuse syndromes. However, today even young children—particularly those who are exposed to repetitive and one-sided physical activity—develop muscle problems. If you spot potential troublemakers early, you can avoid a lot of pain.

Am I Too Old to Heal My Muscles?

My dad is eighty-eight years old. He does not think of muscle pain as a problem. "Don't worry about it," he says, "the muscles heal themselves. It is built into them." His frozen shoulder healed after a fall a couple of years ago. "The pain gradually disappeared," he says. "I did not do anything." But that's not quite true.

My dad walks every day, forty-five minutes in the morning and again in the evening. He skies, he sails, he dives, and he swims, and he refused to give it up as he aged. His shoulder pain healed itself because he moved. His shoulder muscles get stretched to their full range of motion many times a day.

—Beth

The energy we see and admire in those of our elders who have practiced a lifetime of healthy living is proof that what we do really makes a difference. These people took care of themselves. But is it too late for those of us who did not?

The reality is that as we get older, our skin loses elasticity and fluidity, and so do our tendons, ligaments, and connective tissue. As we age, our basic metabolic rate decreases. This means we burn fat more slowly and put on weight, which in turn results in flabby arms, loss of muscle mass, and more.

Muscles atrophy with age. However, this atrophy predominantly affects the fast-fiber types (type II), which are only 15 to 20 percent of the muscle fibers in the body! So while these power-type fibers definitely lose mass and power with age, the rest of the muscle fibers, the slow-fibers (type I) are not affected very much by the aging process. These are the endurance-type fibers, which respond very well to strength training.

(People who perform endurance exercise develop large numbers of these fibers, whereas those who do weightlifting exercises develop large numbers of the power-type fibers.) So, the good news is that significant strength gain and muscle healing are possible in elderly people.

Through the normal aging process, the number of small blood vessels that supply our tissue capillaries decreases, and our blood vessels tend to constrict more easily. This means that it takes more effort for the heart to push blood through our blood vessels. Therefore, the circulation can become reduced; yet to heal your muscle pain, you need blood flow.

However, when you build strength in your endurance-type muscle fibers, you substantially increase the number of capillaries in your muscles as long as you keep exercising. Exercising can also increase the flow of blood to your muscles by 80 percent. When you massage and stretch your muscles, you also increase blood flow significantly. The ability to control chronic pain by exercising is the same in both young and old people.

It is never too late, too hard, or too complicated to heal muscle pain. Our bodies, young or old, have the capacity to heal wounds, rebuild tissue, enhance the blood circulation, and regain lost strength!

CHAPTER 4

Taking the Burden off Your Muscles

I wanted to improve my posture because I experienced repeated painful muscle spasms in my upper back and neck. Over the years I had developed a habit of holding my upper back hunched a little forward. When I tried to straighten it, I found that I simply could not do it. I was unable to move my shoulders and upper back backward. I blamed it on my age and concluded that the vertebrae of my upper spine had become calcified and unable to move. However, my physical therapist said he would prove me wrong. Despite my disbelief and apprehension, he skillfully arched the row of vertebrae of my stiff-as-a-board upper back into a complete and full backward range of motion.

There was really nothing wrong with my spine. In contrast, my chronically tight chest muscles had pulled my upper body forward, making a posture change simply impossible. My overstretched and weakened back muscles had suffered for years. My therapist repeated the backward bending exercise during each session. I started stretching the chest muscles on my own. Soon, I could lift my chest and straighten my back. Now I breathe freer, stand taller, and, most importantly, my neck feels more mobile and comfortable. I no longer get the back spasms I used to have during stress.

—Chris

Our muscles are designed to work perfectly in balance, yet we repeatedly upset this balance and then wonder why our muscles scream in pain. Simply straightening the upper back and neck brings the joints back into a balanced position, giving the neck and back muscles enough of a break to help restore normal blood circulation.

Although we cannot see our joints and muscles and how they carry the weight of the body and balance the bones, we can certainly learn to be aware when they are not doing so. For example, if you sit and look straight ahead at a computer screen, without bending your neck, your bones carry the weight of your head and your neck muscles can relax. However, the moment you lean a little forward—as usually happens when the monitor is placed too low—you create a burden for your neck and upper back muscles. The weight of the head that they now must carry has increased. If your head weighs 8 pounds and is held 3 inches forward of the center of gravity, your head now weighs 24 pounds. The head has not gained weight, of course, but due to the effect of gravity, the weight that your neck muscles must support is multiplied by three.

This is not something we are much aware of. Still, it is a fact that leaning or bending any part of our body away from the center of gravity adds more weight that the muscles must carry. Positioning your joints so that the weight of your body parts is close to the center of gravity causes the bones to carry the weight, rather than the muscles. This is alignment.

Aligning Your Body

Your starting position for any exercise

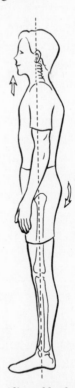

- Stand normally.
- Place your feet parallel, about a fist's width apart, with your weight evenly distributed. Breathe in deeply once and exhale slowly.
- While breathing in again, lift your chest as if it were gently being pulled up toward the ceiling by the collarbone. Continue to lift until you feel your shoulders relax and fall into a natural posture by themselves. Exhale.
- Tighten your buttocks and tuck your tailbone under just a little, keeping the natural curve in your lower back. (Be careful not to tilt your hips too far backward.) Keep your chest lifted.
- Make your neck long and tuck your chin in just a little. Try to breathe comfortably in this new position.

Aligned body
posture

You can think of this as lengthening and stretching your spine, increasing the distance between your collarbone and the tailbone.

The spine has an optimal curve in the upper, middle, and lower back that, when aligned properly, carries the weight of the head, shoulders, and upper body in the best way possible.

Taking advantage of the joints' ability to balance the body lifts the load off your muscles. The difference this makes when it becomes a habit can be immense! The illustration below shows where the line should pass through your joints when your body is aligned and balanced.

Deviation in any direction from the centerline adds stress to the muscles; conversely, any position centering around this line takes the stress away.

It can be helpful to use this as a model even though it is rare for anyone to be perfectly aligned.

Your Muscles Adapt

If you are like most people, you have put your body posture out of alignment in many ways. This is normal. However, your muscles have the ability to adapt and change. They can increase and decrease in strength, length, and size. Over time, they adjust to whatever posture you choose, often struggling to make up for a less-than-ideal alignment. Suddenly attempting to straighten up to achieve a perfect posture can, therefore, be frustrating. Your muscles have a length well suited to your old posture and will not accept the new position right away. But eventually they will. Thanks to your body's ability to learn and adapt, it will soon adjust itself. Don't be surprised if trying to change your posture feels exhausting even though it is not heavy exercise. Even small muscle movements, when unaccustomed, can be tiring.

Once you get used to being aware of how joints and muscles work together you will notice when your muscles are struggling, which enables you to relieve them by simply adjusting your position.

Paying Attention to the Other Side (of the Bending Joint)

If one side of a scale is too heavy, we simply add weight to the other side to restore balance. The muscles, arranged in pairs of opposites, require a balanced load, like a scale. You can think of the muscles on either side of a moving joint as one long muscle. This is not anatomically correct, but is it correct according to muscle dynamics. Everything you do on one side, such as contract or stretch, conversely affects the muscle on the other side.

For example, bending your body forward contracts the muscles in the front, your chest and abdominal muscles, and thus necessarily stretches the muscles in your back. Therefore, contracting one muscle causes the muscle on the opposite side to be stretched for as long as the contraction lasts. Now consider the situation of your back muscles during a long day of bending over your desk.

If you have bent forward for a long time, it is not enough just to straighten up to restore muscle balance. The muscles that have been stretched now need to fully contract. Thus, what you need to do is bend backward for a full range of motion! This way your back muscles get fully contracted, which makes up for the overstretching.

To stay healthy, the muscles must be allowed to contract and relax alternately. Each is equally important. Without contracting they become weak and vulnerable to injury, and without relaxing they neither get sufficient nutrients nor rid their fibers of waste products.

Performing the opposite action by relieving the hardworking front and strengthening the overstretched back has a great relieving effect. The same applies to both sides of the body.

Quick Relief for Tense Back Muscles

Your back muscles are often stretched for long hours as you bend forward while working. To restore balance, gently contract these tense muscles as follows:

- Assume the starting position, (buttocks are tucked in). Place one (or both) arms across the small of your back and lean your upper body back over your arm.
- Start with your arm all the way down on your hip bones. Bend backward. Move your arm up a bit at a time, bending over it as you go. Continue up as far as you can reach. Feel the back bending in many different places as the abdominal muscles lengthen completely. Remember to breathe.
- Do this as often as you can during your workday.

By reversing the situation—doing the exact opposite—you relieve both muscles or muscle groups of tension and restore the balance between them.

If you do this consistently and routinely as you work, taking into consideration the positions in which you hold different parts of your body for long periods of time, you might find that you end up with less and less muscular pain. You are now working with the muscular system and not against it. It is actually a very natural thing to do in response to tightness and strain.

Analyze Your Daily Activities

We are often forced to work in positions that put our bodies out of alignment. For obvious reasons, we cannot avoid these positions altogether, but we can provide periodic relief to our joints and muscles.

Imagine a tower of stacked soda cans on the verge of toppling over. Wouldn't you instinctively rush to restore it to balance? If you were able to see when your bones, joints, and muscles were similarly out of balance, you would probably react the same way. You can. By making a simple, systematic analysis of your daily activities, you can then make a habit of instantly restoring balance as it gets disrupted during your day. Applying this kind of logical thinking is an important step on the path to freeing your muscles from pain.

First and foremost on the path to restoring balance is discovering what you are doing during the day to cause your pain. Focus on identifying one-sided activities that you engage in during the day for prolonged periods of time. Ask yourself questions such as:

• Am I bending my hips more than I am straightening them? (For example, do I sit or bend over for long hours?)

Quick Relief for Tight Hip Muscles

If you sit on a chair for long hours, your front hip muscles are contracted for as long as you sit. Merely standing up is not enough to restore balance between the muscles on both sides of your hips (front and back).

• Stand up. In the starting position, place your hands on your hips. Transfer weight to your left foot with the body still balanced. Keep the body upright and the buttocks tucked in. Slide your right foot back along the floor, moving only the leg, until your toes are bent and your leg is straight.
• Now slowly bend your trunk backward from the hip, lengthening the area that is contracted when you sit. Take your time to

feel the deep muscles inside and in front of the hip being stretched. Take your time to discover the movement of these deep muscles.
- Do the left side as well. Do this often during breaks.

- Am I bending my neck, upper back, or lower back forward more than backward during the day? (For example, do I sit with my head and upper back hunched forward over a desk? Do I bend over to work on the ground, to care for a person in bed, to play a musical instrument, or to change a baby on a table?)
- Am I tilting my head, neck, upper back, or lower back more to one side than to the other? (For example, do I cradle the phone between my ear and shoulder while doing something else with my hands?)
- Am I holding my shoulders tensed forward more than I am letting them move backward during the day? (Do I tense my shoulders this way due to stress and nervousness?)
- Am I contracting the muscles that bend my hip (hip flexors) unevenly? (For example, do I frequently sit cross-legged, with my upper body tilted to one side?)
- Am I turning my upper body more to one side than the other during the workday? (For example, do I hold my body in awkward and twisted positions for extended periods of time, such as in building, painting, or doing repair work?)
- Am I holding my hand in a power grip (as in grasping tools) more than I am straightening my fingers and wrist?

Quick Stretch Relief for Painful Elbows

If you bend (curl) your fingers for long hours, to restore balance:

- Lift your arm straight out in front of you, palm facing down. Bend your wrist by pointing the fingers toward the ceiling. With the other hand, pull your hand and fingers toward your body. Feel the stretch along the palm side of the forearm all the way to the elbow. Do the other arm.
- Also stretch the other side of the forearm with the arm in the same position as above. Make a fist. With the other hand reach around the fist and pull it toward the inside of your forearm. Likewise, feel the stretch along the backside of the forearm.

• Am I turning my feet, knees, hips, and legs more inward than out-ward, or vice versa? (For example, do I turn my foot outward or inward to step on a pedal, or while standing? Do I keep my knees, or one knee, turned out or in while I work?)

• Am I bending my arm at the elbow more than I am straightening it? (For example, do I do desk or any other kind of work in front of the body with bent arms?)

• Am I turning my forearm and palm over more than I'm turning them up? (For example, do I use a keyboard?)

• Am I bending my knees more than I'm straightening them? (For example, do I sit or kneel for long periods of time at work?)

These are merely a few examples of questions you should be asking yourself as you build muscle and body awareness. Continue to ask these and many more relevant questions. Expand your examination to include leisure activities. For each activity, ask yourself:

- Have I caused chronic uneven muscle usage by developing some muscles or muscle groups more than others?
- How can I restore balance by reversing activities, doing the opposite, stretching the side that was contracted and contracting the side that was stretched?

Tightness and pain are the way our muscles try to accommodate our choice of posture and muscle usage. Paying attention to pain and tightness and adjusting your positions so as to relieve discomfort when it appears is the easiest way to deal with them.

You might get the impression that muscles are fragile, since you have to watch your posture so carefully and adjust your position to avoid hurt-ing them. But muscles are not fragile at all. They have extraordinary capac-ity for change: the ability to adapt and recover from abuse and to build strength. When you interfere with the balanced way that muscles work with each other, however, they adapt in order to continue to function, which results in pain and discomfort.

Muscle Jobs

The muscular system is designed to enable us to move freely, to perform at once powerful, heavy-duty tasks and tiny, precise motor movements. All muscles participate in the system as a whole, but each single muscle also has its own unique job to perform.

Most of us pay little attention to a particular muscle until it hurts. Then we suddenly become painfully aware of its location and its job, which the muscle may now refuse to perform. But if we get to know about what stresses a muscle before it hurts, it may never hurt at all. We will notice in time to take preventive action.

Getting to know the muscles that perform the easily recognizable movements you most appreciate is a good introduction to understanding the basics of your muscular system. And it's not as hard as you might think. Even if a muscle performs many jobs at the same time, each has a primary job that you can use to identify the muscle. Bending the knee, for example, is the primary job of the hamstrings. You can easily feel these working in the back of your thigh. Lifting the arm is the main job of the muscle that covers your shoulder, the deltoid. Knowing a muscle's job is the key to verifying that it is healthy and functioning properly.

Muscle Balance—What Is It?

If you discover that the muscles that bend your hip are much tighter and, perhaps, stronger than those that straighten the hip, there is an imbalance in your hip muscles. Sometimes an imbalance is due to lack of strength balance between a group of muscles that do the same job. The key to removing muscle pain is to untangle such imbalances. It is easy, once you look more closely at how the muscles work together.

In a muscle group, each muscle has a different role to play. Becoming familiar with these roles can seem confusing at first, but there is a great reward: You will be able to understand muscle dynamics and begin to see and understand the origins of your pain and how it developed. You can then set up a logical strategy for avoiding, preventing, and healing it in the future.

Depending on which motion you execute, your muscles can play the role of the:

Primary Mover (Agonist).   This is the muscle that is mainly responsible for the movement at a joint. For example, the muscle that bends the hand at the wrist (wrist flexor) is the primary mover for this motion.

Opposing Muscle (Antagonist).   This is the muscle that executes the exact opposite motion of the primary mover. For example, the muscle that lifts the hand at the wrist (wrist extensor) is the opposing muscle to the wrist flexor for the motion of bending the hand at the wrist.

Assisting Muscles (Synergists).   The primary mover seldom does its job alone. The assisting muscles support the primary mover in its motion. For example, the muscles that bend the fingers are assisting muscles to the wrist flexors because they also help with the bending of the hand at the wrist.

The muscles do not work alone but in pairs and groups: pairs of opposites, pairs of like muscles (twins), and groups of supporting muscles.

Pairs of Opposites

When you identify one muscle and its job, there is always another muscle carrying out the opposite motion in a dependable and balanced fashion. The primary and opposing movers form a pair of opposites.

For example, the front and back thigh muscles work together as a pair. When you bend your knee, the hamstrings are the primary movers and the quads are the opposing movers. During one single movement, such as the bending of the knee, both muscles are affected: one is stretched while the other contracts. If the usage patterns of the two sides differ significantly, as when only the quads get a lot of strengthening while the hamstrings barely get any, the two sides will not work well together. A rule of thumb is:

What we make our muscles do on one side of a joint always affects the muscles on the opposite side.

Primary and opposing muscles have clearly identifiable separate jobs, yet are so interdependent that they almost function as one. If a primary mover becomes tight and stays shortened, a common muscle response to overuse injury, the opposing muscle will also become injured, because it has to adapt to the situation by becoming longer than natural.

The interaction between the pairs of opposite muscles is crucial for any movement to happen. We tend to take this for granted. For example, when you bend your body backward, the contracting back muscles are making it happen. At the same time, although you do not notice it, the abdominal muscles in the front automatically relax.

But imagine what happens when the opposing muscle does not relax, but stays contracted! You would be unable to bend backward at all. Very often our muscles only relax partially. The movement—in this case bending backward—is similarly only partially completed. Most of us have some muscles that do not move to full range. When we do attempt a full range of motion, there are tight muscles inhibiting the movement. By understanding and taking control of these functions, you can skillfully find such muscles, bring them back to full range, and experience great relief.

Always Restore Balance

Any time you feel tightness in an area of your body:

- Stretch the tight muscles to the full range of motion.
- Also stretch the muscles on the other side of the joint, the opposing muscles.

It is obvious that your muscles work while you move, but if you could see exactly when your muscles move, you might be surprised. After doing knee-bending exercises, your front thigh muscles often get very sore. This is because during knee bending they contract both while you straighten the knees, which is their primary job, and while you bend, to stabilize the bending process so you do not fall to the ground (see "Eccentric Contraction," Chapter 7). Therefore, there is a double load on these muscles during knee bending: while you go down and also as you come up.

Muscles not only make us move, they also make us stop moving. Thanks to the opposing muscle, it is possible for us to stop when we are in motion. It immediately contracts, holding the body back.

For example, if you are about to set an item on a table and then change your mind, you can stop the motion in midair. The job of the muscle that straightens the arm, the triceps, is canceled by the action of the muscle on the other side of the upper arm, the biceps, because it contracts while you are in the process of straightening your arm. During any movement—running, walking, or just moving your body—if you contract the opposing muscle with enough force, you will stop the movement. Injuries often occur during sudden, abrupt movements when the opposing muscle lacks the strength to handle the extra load of stopping your movement.

Remember: When the primary mover contracts, the opposing muscle relaxes. The primary mover and the opposing muscle can also contract simultaneously to stabilize the body. Opposing muscles bring the moving body to a halt.

Pairs of Alike Muscles (Twins)

Because the body is symmetrical you will always find a muscle on one side of the spine, left and right, that is an exact copy of and carries out precisely the same job as one on the other side. They have the same strength and length. For example, the muscles that bend the left hand are exactly like those that bend the right hand. The left and right legs' hamstrings are exactly like each other, like twins. The muscles are arranged in perfect symmetry to the left and right side of the spine, thus creating balance.

Through our movements and habits, however, we often create imbalance between these muscles. The twin that is tighter will pull toward its side and bring the alignment away from the center of gravity. When you bend to the side, the opposing muscle (the twin) provides resistance and holds you back so you do not tip over.

Many people are told that they have one leg that is shorter than the other without actually having a skeletal abnormality. Very often, the muscles on one side of the body, especially those muscles that bend the torso to the side, have become unevenly tight. A certain strength balance within the group is required for the muscles to function without pain.

A Group of Supporting Muscles

If a muscle has been weakened by injury or abuse, you are not out of luck. There is a surrounding muscle group that will support and take over if your weakened muscle fails to do its job fully. The muscles in this group have separate primary jobs of their own, but also have helping functions with other muscles. They consist of a primary mover and its assisting muscles.

Checking for Symmetry

- Looking in the mirror, notice if one collarbone, shoulder, or hipbone seems higher than the other.
- Determine which muscle is causing this to happen (look up the muscle jobs in Chapter 9). Start stretching this muscle. Persist until you see a change.

Therefore, when your hurt muscles have healed, you are improving your overall muscular system if you also check the condition of the supporting muscles, those that helped out. Often, we do all the right things—stretch, strengthen, and treat the muscle that was hurt, and even take time off work—yet after we go back to our regular activity, the symptom soon reappears. The reason could be that the supporting muscles are still tight.

After Injury

- After muscle pain or an injury and after having been checked by a physician, treat, stretch, and strengthen the hurt muscle.
- Look up the assisting movers that belong to the group of your hurt muscle.
- Treat, stretch, and strengthen these supporting muscles as well.

The interactions within and among muscle groups teach us that treating only one muscle does not fix the problem. Often pain seems to extend over a large area of the body. Tightness in one muscle initially leads to tightness in its assisting, opposing, and twin muscles. Unevenly tight neck muscles can lead to unevenly tight upper back muscles and unevenly tight hip muscles. The whole body can become lopsided. By making sure we treat the whole muscle group, we eliminate the most common reason for spreading a muscle problem: involving more and more muscles in the pain cycle.

Maintaining the balance between these factors is, in a nutshell, what takes the stress and burden off our muscles so health and well-being can return. You can, during your day, reverse the impact on your body of one-sided movement and habitual muscle usage, and relieve your muscles of pain as it occurs.

CHAPTER 5

Starting the Healing Process

I put my shoes on and stumbled out on my morning walk. It was early: my body was not ready to move, and my shoulders hurt! But there was nothing new about that; I always had a dull ache in them. That morning I paid attention to my shoulders and arms. I had never noticed how little my arms moved while I walked. I realized that to avoid feeling the pain in my shoulders, I had not allowed my arms to move. The doctor who examined my shoulders told me that I would have less pain if I moved and exercised more, which surprised me because I had a habit of exercising regularly. I now started deliberately swinging my arms back and forth as I walked. It was not a pleasurable sensation. After a couple of days, however, my shoulders felt different. It seemed to me that the pain had started to taper off. I expanded the motion with the shoulders; folding my arms across my back as I walked was especially painful. I instinctively started rubbing and massaging my shoulders. This helped. I increased the massage and started pressing on the bones on top of and around the shoulders as I walked. I realized I was now chasing the pain. Wherever I found it I pushed, pressed, moved, and massaged. Healing happened over a couple of weeks, slowly but surely, finally leaving my shoulders pain-free, night and day.

—Elisabeth

Pain like that just described, which disappears when the area is moved and stimulated, is the kind of unnecessary pain we hold in our bodies. It is quite an amazing experience to feel pain leaving areas that have been hurting for a long time. Such pain, though, is widespread and much more abundant in our hips, shoulders, neck, lower back, thighs, knees, forearms, elbows, and wrists than we are aware of, producing aching, fluid-filled, inflamed tissue along with tense muscles and restricted joints. Although we can dull the symptoms for a while by using anti-inflammatory pain relievers, there are much better routes open to us that promote healing and lasting relief.

This is exactly what manual treatment aims to do, and it is also why we feel so good after being treated by physical and massage therapists, who use their hands rather than medication. Each has his or her unique method of treatment, although they are all taught specific standard techniques to facilitate movement at the joints, reduce tension in muscles and tendons, and increase the circulation. Some have developed extraordinary abilities over years of understanding the body through their hands.

It is a gift to receive such treatment. The results, however, also offer us a firsthand demonstration of our body's own pain-relieving and healing capacity, a powerful tool that each of us can benefit from utilizing.

Discover Your Tools and Develop Your Technique

Therapists use their hands differently than we do. They "listen" to the bones, tissue, and muscles, using their fingers knowingly and purposefully to relieve pain. You also can learn to understand the language of your body.

Take a look at your hand. You use your fingers all the time and you know what a grip is; however, focusing your attention on your fingers as massage and pain-relieving tools is somewhat different.

Your strong thumb is an excellent worker for the purpose of palpating, sensing, rubbing, and massaging what is under the skin. With the large pad, which has a lot of sensory nerves in and under the skin, you can sense, push, press, and rub into muscle, tendon, vessels, bones, and soft and hard tissue. After a while, your thumb will develop an awareness of the differences. Try this, for example, on your forearm: With your elbow bent (forearm held across your abdomen), place your thumb on the bones of your elbow and feel their hardness. As you move down the arm, be aware of the difference between soft and hard areas, the movable muscle bellies and the stringy cords of tendons farther down the arm. You will need to press in and move the tissue across the arm to feel the differences.

The second, third, and fourth fingers together make a sensitive three-finger pad. If you hold them tightly together you can use them as a solid and strong tool for pressing into the tissue and rubbing it. Using your thumb and three-finger pad together gives you a means by which to pinch, rub, grab, push, massage, pump, and knead the muscles and the tissue, all of which stimulate blood circulation. Also, the ball of your thumb together with the three-finger pad gives you another good grip for pumping motion when that is needed. To achieve even more pressure, use your knuckles to rub and massage up and down your thighs, legs, and arms. To do this, make a fist and use the middle row of knuckles. Even your elbow can effectively be used to apply pressure on areas you can reach.

Before you start using the different methods available to increase blood circulation and relieve pain in your muscles, make sure you consult a doctor in case your pain stems from an injury or a disease that requires treatment other than normal tissue and muscle activity. Here are some techniques to try:

Rubbing

Rubbing tissue that hurts is an instinctive reaction. When a child has been hurt, parents rub the site of the injury. You most likely perform this natural action without registering it when you hurt. Rubbing, which creates friction and movement in the tissue, is one of the principal manual tools with which to help rid muscles of pain. But how can such a seemingly unsophisticated activity cause pain to go away?

When you rub, move, and massage, you apply pressure on everything from blood and lymphatic vessels to microscopic pores in the tissue that fluids are moved through. The pressure from your fingers affects the vessels and pores. You can think about it as a way of momentarily holding the fluids back, like in a dam, and when you let go, blood and other fluids rush through at a faster speed. Although this happens at a microscopic level, the effect is similar. This increased circulation helps to drain fluid accumulation, promote exchange between fluid compartments, and stimulate the cleaning process. Waste products are removed more efficiently, which helps restore chemical balance.

Any kind of movement will achieve some of this—walking, stretching, or massage—but by intentionally rubbing and massaging the skin and the tissue above and around the painful spot, you are activating the circulation.

Cross-Fiber Massage

When you rub and massage across the fibers, for example, across your thigh instead of along its length, you help move your flesh in a direction that normal body movement usually does not provide. Cross-fiber massage, therefore, causes most needed motion and friction when the fibers and tissue are denied renewed nutrients and oxygen.

When you massage across the muscle fibers you also more effectively help loosen up adhesions. The muscle functions better, which helps the muscle fibers and tissues to function normally.

(For all Circulation Aid boxes, see muscle illustrations in Chapter 9.)

Circulation Aid 1

Tendon Massage (Muscle: Pectoralis Major)

- Starting about three inches from the tip of your shoulder, feel and palpate along the underside of your collarbone.
- Press in with your three-finger pads and move your fingers sideways back and forth, in tiny circles in a rubbing fashion.
- Feel the difference between the bone and the tendon.
- Move slowly toward the breastbone, and right where you feel the collarbone ends, follow the breastbone down. Feel the bumps of each new rib where this muslce attaches. It is common to feel very sore here.
- Follow slowly, rib by rib, down to where the rib cage arches out.
- Remember the attachment on your arm, too. Using your thumb, rub up and down the front of the arm right below the shoulder.

End with a slow shoulder stretch (Chapter 12) to help wash away wastes. Palpating and reviving the tendons of all key muscles and noting your individual problem areas will give you a unique healing technique you can utilize anytime and anywhere.

Circulation Aid 2

Muscle Belly Massage (Muscle: Triceps Brachii)

- Start on the back of your upper arm, about three inches down from the top of your shoulder.
- Press in with your three-finger pad and run it across the soft area from the back to the side and back again.
- Feel the textures of the long fiber bundles.
- Move down a little at the time, rubbing cross-fiber until you are three inches from the elbow.
- End with a slow elbow stretch (See Chapter 12).

Cross-fiber massaging the bellies of all key muscles will enable you to skillfully supply extra blood flow to your individual painful muscles anytime, anywhere.

"Dragging" the Tissue and Twisting It

The more motion you create, the more effectively you will stimulate the circulation and the less likely it will be that your tissue develops problems from lack of oxygen. Moving whole sheets of tissue can be very effective at causing motion in the many layers right under your skin, where there is an abundance of blood vessels.

Circulation Aid 3

Moving the Tissue (Thigh and Leg Muscles)

- Encircle your thigh firmly with both hands. While you press in, drag the soft tissue first one way and then the other.
- As you do this, move your hands up and down the thigh.
- Next, work up and down the leg and down over the knee and the lower leg, and get a full-leg circulation rush.

You can do this wherever you can reach. You can drag the tissue around your waist and over your shoulder across your lower back and buttocks the same way and give yourself a whole-body circulation boost.

Skin Rolling

Another great way to increase blood flow around your hurting muscle is to roll the skin between your fingers to create extra friction and motion there. The layers of tissue right under the skin are rich in blood vessels, sensory nerves, and tissue fluids.

You can verify the effect of applying pressure to and rubbing your skin. Locate a spot where your skin looks pale, press there for a couple of seconds, and let go. You will see that the previously pale area is suddenly red and flushed. The pressure from your fingers caused your blood vessels to immediately widen out (dilate) to rush blood to the area where your pressure had caused what your body interprets as an "emergency" situation—lack of blood flow.

Circulation Aid 4

Skin Rolling (Muscle: Wrist Extensors)

- Hold the skin of your forearm between your thumb and three-finger pad.

- Lift up and roll the skin, moving it like a wave across the arm.
- Push and drag the thumb against the skin.

End with a slow stretch (see Chapter 12).

Applying Pressure

Think back to a time when you were hit really hard. You might have grabbed the hurt spot and held onto it as hard as you could. You were putting pressure on the painful spot. You did it instinctively, but you can also do it deliberately to reduce pain. Applying deliberate and sustained pressure (for a short period of time) on tendons and muscles is a method used in many different forms by therapists.

The earliest known form of acupuncture involved applying pressure to the painful area of the body. Later, this developed into a healing system. A common acupuncture technique is one in which the practitioner punctures certain areas called Ah Shi points (meaning: Ah, yes! That's where it hurts) and thus relieves pain. These acupuncture points correspond closely to the points at which the nerves enter the muscle (motor point). Today a method used by massage and physical therapists of treating certain tender areas in the muscles is based on the premise that there are certain points (trigger points) in the muscles. When treated, they relieve the muscle of pain. It is thought that these points are areas of tiny spasms that go away when you apply pressure to them and massage and stretch the area. Yet another method that uses the application of pressure on sore spots to relieve pain is the one in which you position a tennis ball under a sore spot in your back, shoulder, or hip. When you let the weight of your body fall on the ball, you experience a firm pressure. Usually you will be told to lie on the tennis ball until the pain recedes. There are a variety of new massage tools on the market, built especially for applying pressure on tender spots.

Circulation Aid 5

Applying Pressure

You can help relieve pain in a very sore area by imitating an instinctive reaction. Grab the sore spot and hold firmly as if you have been suddenly hit. Hold it for a couple of seconds. Fresh blood will rush to the pained area upon release.

What does applying pressure do? It functions like rubbing does, only more so. Simply put, it increases the circulation by creating a buildup of pressure in the vessels carrying fluids, causing the fluids to rush through with greater speed when you let go. You can experiment with different ways of applying pressure and experience it working.

Pumping the Tissue

Pressing on tendons and muscles, then letting go at intervals, functions like a pump to the circulation. If you have a sore muscle or tendon attachment, it can be very helpful to use this pumping technique to stimulate the circulation to the area. When the blood is rushing through there is less pain, and you may be more able to gently stretch the muscle.

Circulation Aid 6

Pumping the Blood Flow (The Hip and Thigh Muscles)

- Put your hands on your leg just above your knee. With short but firm pumping motions, press and let go in a steady rhythm. Move up the thigh about an inch at a time.
- Put both hands on the outside of your leg, right above the knee. Press and release as above, moving up the thigh all the way to the top of the thighbone. Continue pumping around this bone. Keep this up until you get a warm sensation as the blood rushes through.

  You can use this technique in any area where you feel tightness and pain.

Stretch and Contract while Applying Pressure

You can also press in on a muscle or tendon deliberately while you move, stretch, and contract, just as the person described at the beginning of this chapter did. This increases the effectiveness of both the massage and the stretch and contraction. When you become skilled in this technique, you have a tool you may come to love in helping your hurt muscles recover.

Circulation Aid 7

Contract While You Apply Pressure (Arm Muscles)

Put your thumb under and the other four fingers on top of your forearm about two inches below the elbow. Hold firmly and press in while you lift your hand, extending the wrist. This motion contracts the wrist and finger muscles at the top of the forearm. You should feel the muscles move under your fingers. Move to the exact spot where there is soreness and repeat this motion several times, releasing the pressure after you lift the wrist.

Stretch While You Apply Pressure

Now press the same spots but this time stretch the muscles instead of contracting them. Bend the hand toward the inside of the forearm, flexing the wrist. (This motion stretches the muscles on top of the forearm.)

Move to the exact spot where there is soreness and press in while you stretch.

Keep in mind that when you press the muscle or tendon, the monitoring system gets involved more actively than during regular stretching and contraction. The length monitors interpret pressing on a muscle as an increase in length. Therefore, you may feel a pulling back inside the fibers stronger than the one experienced during regular stretching. This tells you to use the technique with care and experiment until you know how your muscles react to your treatment. It also has the positive effect of speeding up all the processes of healing.

Putting pressure on a muscle or tendon while you contract it increases the pressure within the muscle, which propels the circulation when you relax. In addition, you affect the tension monitors, which interpret the pressure as an increase in tension and may alert the fibers to relax the muscle. Some therapists treating muscles that are unable to relax intentionally put pressure right where the muscle fibers widen out and become the tendon, which is where the tension monitors are located, and achieve a complete relaxation of the muscle. This is also done during stretching and contraction. You can gently try out these methods with your own muscles.

Breathing Life into Hurt Muscles

When therapists work on the tissue and muscles they find that while patients start to relax and breathe normally, which means deeply, they can feel the tissue change under their hands. It gives in more easily, and moves and stretches more willingly. It is easy to fall prey to shallow breathing during times of stress. Sometimes we can be under stress all day long.

Circulation Aid 8

Breathing Exercises

- Place a wide plastic straw between your lips and close them tight around it. Breathe in through your nose, filling your abdomen (not your chest) with air as deeply as you can. Do not stop inhaling until the need to exhale initiates exhalation by itself.

- Very slowly, let the air out through the straw. Don't stop exhaling until you must inhale. The resisted exhalation prevents your chest from collapsing like a punctured balloon, giving your diaphragm muscle a controlled motion.

You can also do this same exercise without a straw, following the same steps. Instead of letting the air out through the straw, you let it seep out through your lips against resistance while you say *fffffffffffff,* resting your teeth lightly on the lower lip. This is an excellent, foolproof breathing exercise you can do anytime and anywhere, instantly relaxing your whole body.

It is hard to change breathing habits because they are a result of life-long habits.

Circulation Aid 9

Yawning

Think of the way you breathe during an early morning stretch after a long night of lying still. Then yawn. This is a model way of breathing through a stretch! Accompanying your stretches with a yawn can shorten the time it takes to heal your muscle by making more oxygen available to the fibers.

Everybody knows how to yawn, which is one of the most effective ways to increase blood flow to your muscles. The act of yawning is said to propel blood into the veins due to changes in pressure inside the thorax during yawning. This speeds up the circulation. Providing extra oxygen to the pain site makes a big difference and reduces adrenaline levels, which also has a calming effect on your system.

Calming Your Tense Muscles

You cannot command your muscles to relax. They just will not do it! Still, there are things you can do. Learning to benefit from the relaxation reflex that is built into your muscles adds very useful tools to your skills. Treatment methods based on these reflexes are used by therapists in many different combinations.

Tense and Relax. This kind of contraction can give you a feeling of a rush of blood flow to the muscle, followed by relaxation. All you do is deliberately tense the muscle and hold it before you let go. Your body does not move. Tension builds within the fibers as you tense (contract) them. Then the fibers are designed to relax for 5 to 10 seconds afterward. As you tense and let go, tense and let go, you pump the circulation and wash toxins out of the muscle. Now your muscle will respond better to massage and stretching.

Circulation Aid 10a

Tense and Relax (Muscles: Calves)

- Focus on the muscles in the back of your lower leg, the calf muscles (placing your hand on the muscle will let you feel the contraction).
- To relax the muscle: Slowly tense this area, but not to the limit. Hold for one second, then relax. Repeat. Relax. End with a yawn.

Circulation Aid 10b

Tense and Relax (Muscles: Shoulders)

- Sit in starting position.
- Slowly tense up one shoulder, taking your time; feel the tension start deep inside the shoulder and spread outward.
- Hold for 10 seconds, then relax.
- Repeat.
- Do this intermittently throughout the day.

Try this with all key muscles and you will soon develop the awareness and ability to control muscle tension wherever and whenever you need it.

Contract a Muscle All the Way.   Contracting a muscle all the way is a method used by therapists to cause the muscle to relax. In this book we call it "giving the muscle what it asks for," which is pulling together—contraction.

Physiologically, your body works this way also. Contracting fully causes an involuntary (reflex) relaxation. The length monitors relax the muscle—that is, they stop firing messages to contract. This is not a complete relaxation, but it provides enough relaxation to make the muscle much more willing to be worked afterwards.

This exercise also makes a very good emergency tool. If you stretched too far too fast, or for any other reason, it might seem as if the muscle is about to pull into a spasm, so give it what it wants immediately and completely—a full, controlled contraction and hold—and most likely it will ease and come out of it.

Contract the Opposing Muscle.   There is yet another relaxation reflex available, designed to prevent muscles from working against each other. One muscle must relax—the opposing muscle—for the main muscle to be able to contract. Remember, the hamstrings relax when the quads contract—they have to! Therapists use several different and sometimes complicated patterns of contraction and relaxation methods built on these two relaxation reflexes. The most important tip to remember is that you can find the opposing muscle and contract it to relax the muscle (primary mover) that is tense. This can seem a little complicated at first, but when you get used to it, this is a very helpful tool to get tense muscles to let go. As you learn the language of the body and sense it at work, with time you will be able to use it to manage the condition of your muscles.

Circulation Aid 11

Contract All the Way (Neck Muscles)

- Start in a sitting position. The couch is perfect for this, as you can support your neck.
- Lean your head backwards a little while lifting your shoulders to meet the back of your neck. Contract all the way (very gently—neck muscles need a slow tempo), hold for a little, and then relax.
- Next, tilt your head to the side and a little backward, also lifting the shoulder, and contract again.

- Repeat in as many directions as you can, bringing your shoulders up to meet the back of the head.
- Take time to notice that the muscle really feels more relaxed. It will: it is made to do exactly that.

Try this with all key muscles.

Circulation Aid 12

Contract the Opposing Muscle (Quads and Hamstrings)

Use this when your quads are tight and will not stretch without great pain.

- While standing, bend your knee lifting heel toward the buttocks, contracting the hamstrings (opposing muscles), and hold for 10 seconds. Relax.
- Immediately stretch your quads (see p. 249).
- Turn it around: While sitting, raise your foot up until your leg is extended straight forward. Contract and hold for 10 seconds. Relax.
- Immediately stretch your hamstrings (see p. 248).

Try this with all key muscles.

The morning after you have worked sore spots, pained tissue, and tight muscles, you are likely to wake up feeling that these spots are even more sore. This is the point at which people say, "I tried it, but it didn't work," and give up. However, by rubbing, moving, and stirring the tissue, you are starting the healing process. Light adhesions between muscle fibers and connective tissue fibers are separated and broken up when you rub them. The tissue often gets a little roughed up, similar to what happens when muscle damage occurs during uncustomary motion and exercise. As a result, irritation and even some inflammation in the area can occur.

PAIN AFTER SELF-TREATMENT?

You are getting better, not worse! It is okay if you feel some more pain after you have started working on a sore area. This is a sign that healing has started. The body's own process includes some swelling, some inflammation, and thus some increased pain. When the body gets to do its job, your pain will go away.

SMALL AREAS OF SWELLING (EDEMA)

When a healthy cell is forced to operate under shortage of fuel from the blood or when it gets crushed during injury and tries to survive, it accumulates fluid. Therefore, tiny areas of swelling (edema) can appear in your muscle fibers, tendons, and tissue. This is a natural process of diluting chemicals inside the cell to maintain chemical balance (homeostasis). Such swelling can be very slight, yet still affect the blood flow in the muscle.

When allowed to remain, the watery content of the cells becomes thicker because of a chemical reaction in the fluid and is now more like a solid obstruction to surrounding blood vessels. The swelling that was produced by lack of blood flow has thus become a cause of lack of blood flow.

Inside each muscle cell, which is like a chemical factory, there is no pain when balance, or homeostasis, exists between the different substances. When swelling develops, it is an attempt by the body to restore the balance. You can bring homeostasis back to your tissue. By aiding the healing blood circulation, you provide the cell with what it needs to restore the lost balance, and your pain goes away.

YOU CAN HELP REDUCE SWELLING

Swelling is continuously reduced during exercise and movement, which helps eliminate the cell's need to accumulate fluid. New nutrients are supplied and a cleaning out of debris occurs. This causes the swelling to vanish over time. Unless your swelling is due to an acute injury, you can help speed up this process by alternately using ice and heat packs. Ice reduces the amount of fluids entering the cell, and heat rushes nutrients to the cell. You can also speed up the healing process by carefully and persistently rubbing and massaging around swollen areas.

What Is Inflammation?

Inflammation is the process of removing debris and dead cells and replacing these with new, living cells.

Low levels of inflammation are a very important and productive stage in healing. Inflamation in itself is not an infection, unless the area has become infected with foreign bacteria. Your body actually benefits from this renewed and stirred-up cleaning and repair activity, which causes increased blood flow and new building of tissue. You should, however, consult your doctor when you experience inflammation and swelling in order to determine the cause.

Swelling has no known value of its own. Even minor swelling can compress blood vessels in both tissue and nerves. Therefore, you want to actively work to get rid of it (see "Using Ice and Heat," below).

Using Ice and Heat

Ice

Painful muscles can feel swollen and warm as inflammation and repair take place. Ice offers a fast way to calm this down. You can apply an ice pack enclosed in a very thin towel, to protect your skin from the freezing cold. Pain is greatly reduced by ice for several reasons: First, the cold constricts the blood vessels, reducing swelling. As a result, pain from pressure caused by swelling is relieved. Further, cold desensitizes the nerve endings, so the pain is not felt as strongly.

Make Your Own Ice Pack

- Crush ice cubes
- Put the crushed ice in a zip-lock bag, making a $\frac{1}{2}''$ thick layer
- Wrap the bag in a thin, damp towel to protect your skin.
- Apply the ice pack on the painful area or use the ice pack to gently massage the area.
- Continue this for 10–15 minutes
- Let it rest for 15 minutes
- Repeat this sequence several times

However, using ice can stiffen the muscles and tissue and therefore contribute to tighter, contracted muscle fibers, again causing pain. Thus, sometimes using ice alone causes more problems.

Heat

After a hot bath, a soak in the hot tub, or a visit to the sauna, your body has a warm and fuzzy feeling and you become relaxed. Heat dilates your blood vessels, fresh blood rushes to your skin, and connective tissue becomes more smooth and willing to let go, making heat a valuable instrument in treating painful muscles.

Heat can positively interfere with the vicious cycle of pain by reducing discomfort and relaxing microspasms. Applying heat to a muscle before you stretch it makes a big difference in its ability to contract and relax. However, heat on painful muscles can also sometimes increase swelling. Therefore, as with ice application, it is not beneficial to use alone.

Make Your Own Heat Pack

- The easiest and fastest way to make a hot pack is to use a long, large sock made of thin cotton fabric.
- Fill it with rice or buckwheat.
- Tie the sock at the end.
- Microwave it for 3 minutes.
- When it is warm, wrap a thin towel around it to protect your skin.
- Hold your hot pack on the painful area for 10 to 15 minutes.
- Remove for 15 minutes.
- Repeat the sequence.

Moist Heat

- Wet a thin towel.
- Wrap it in two layers around your heated homemade hot pack.
- Apply it to the painful area.

This simple homemade hot pack will stay warm for 15 to 20 minutes. You can reheat it in the microwave when it starts cooling off.

For Best Results, Use Both Ice and Heat

Apply ice massage for 10 minutes to your painful area, then soothe it with the hot pack for another 10 minutes. Repeat this sequence several times and you will achieve the best results.

Learning to alternate the use of heat and ice in cooperation with your health care professional gives you new tools with which to manipulate your system into letting go of pain.

CHAPTER 6

What Is Stretching?

A couple of years ago I learned something about muscle and tissue healing that changed the way I treat my body. I was working on my garage roof, cleaning out the gutter. Suddenly I slipped and fell six feet onto a hard wooden patio. When I came to my senses, I realized that I had hurt my shoulder. I could not move or stand up because of the pain. I was sure that something was terribly wrong.

The doctor told me that I had a separated shoulder, a condition in which ligaments, muscle, and tissue are severely stretched and hurt and the shoulder bone is displaced, not fully dislocated. Nothing was broken. No ligaments were torn. X-ray and MRI results proved that surgery was not necessary, so the doctor sent me home with some stretching exercises to do. I stared at him in disbelief. I had never been in this much pain! Breathing, moving, everything caused a lot of pain. Yet my doctor told me that the more I moved, the sooner the pain would go away. I waited a couple of weeks because I was still in severe pain, but then my doctor told me it was time to start stretching my shoulder gently. The fact that it hurt me to move was not alarming to him. He told me to work through the pain. I worried about this, but I trusted his experience and knowledge. I worked through the pain, against my own instincts to remain immobile. It was not hard once I understood that this pain was not harmful. It was simply recovery pain.

My shoulder recovered faster than anyone expected for someone my age. The pain eased steadily, and my collarbone, which had been sticking up oddly, slowly moved back into place. Today I have no pain in my shoulder and none of the common lifelong signs of an injury. My shoulder looks different, and it will never be completely normal, but the problem is solely cosmetic. I have no pain or stiffness.

—Mark

What Is Stretching and Why Is It Good for Us?

Strictly speaking, stretching a muscle means moving the two tendon attachment sites of the muscle further apart so that the muscle belly fibers are lengthened. A muscle can't stretch itself; it must be stretched. How can this simple movement release such a chain reaction of positive events in our muscles and bodies? The easiest way to answer this question is to look at what exactly is being stretched. It's the muscle, right? But it is more than that. When we stretch a muscle, we also stretch everything inside and around that muscle, including the connective tissue surrounding the muscles, the tissue wrapping the tiny muscle fibers, the tissue around the nerves and blood vessels, the nerves and vessels themselves, and everything else in there.

So what happens when all of this is stretched? The circulation of fluids in and around the muscle, including pain-relieving and nutritious blood, is immediately activated and facilitated when we start to stretch. Lubricating fluid is exchanged in the collagen fibers of tendons, ligaments, and connective tissue as you hold these fibers stretched out. When you relax after the stretch, fresh blood rushes into the fibers and replaces waste products with nutrients.

Also, because there are plenty of sensory nerves in the connective tissue, muscle fibers, nerves, and blood vessels, messages are sent to the central nervous system whenever any changes occur. Therefore, by stretching you start a whole orchestra of message-generating activity. This wakes up and exercises your nervous system. The length monitors report changes in the length of fibers in the muscle belly as the muscle lengthens, and the tension monitors in the tendons report on changes there. The nerve endings in the tissue report changes in metabolism (for example, waste product overload), and receptors in the joints report movements in their arena. Your nervous system needs to be exercised as much as your muscles.

The tangible result of all these internal processes is that you start to sense energy flowing back into your system, pain is reduced, and you relax more and feel better both during and after stretching. Stretching also causes a lasting change for the better.

Nothing can be permanent in the body, since everything is constantly changing. However, the muscle fibers will stay at the length you have trained them to be unless you actively do something to change them back again. After you have been stretching for a while, you will suddenly notice that the muscle you were working on has changed. The muscle fibers have literally become longer! Technically speaking, the tissue around the muscle fibers has adapted to the new length by creating additional tiny fiber sections (sarcomeres) to fill the space inside the muscle.

Let us say that you have neck pain and have started stretching your neck. It is pretty amazing to realize that your neck range has increased so that instead of only being able to turn your head straight to the side, you can actually turn enough to look behind you without twisting your upper body. This is quite an improvement, not only for your neck muscles, but for your entire body. Because you no longer need to twist to see behind you, you have removed excess stress on your upper, middle, and lower back. The rotation of the joint located between the two vertebrae at the top of the spine (C1 and C2) is finally allowed to work at its full range!

Arriving at the point when you can turn your head more, reach further, or bend lower with less discomfort is possible thanks to the same adaptability that caused your muscle to shorten and tighten in the first place. Just as you probably didn't notice your muscle tightening until the pain set in, you may not sense your muscle lengthening until you notice your increased range of motion and ability (not to mention the absence of pain!). By stretching, however, you have achieved even more.

- You have had an impact on your body alignment, because minor changes in muscle length adjust the way the muscles hold and align the body.
- You have started adjusting the muscle balance in your body, because a change in one muscle's length affects the length of other muscles in the muscle group.
- You have improved the health of your joints, because these are supplied with nutritious fluid and become stronger when you move.
- You have improved the quality of the connective tissue in the areas you have stretched, because the collagen fibers get strengthened.

Learning to initiate and take charge of these influential events in your body will help you develop an attitude of challenge instead of defeat toward your muscle pain. You can do a lot to change your condition. Stretching is only one thing, but it is most central to finding relief.

Stretching Intelligently

When we consult a physical therapist, we are likely to be sent home with a set of stretches and strengthening exercises to carry out between appointments. And all too often, we end up doing nothing between appointments, or even quitting treatment altogether. This chapter introduces you to the principles behind stretching and the everyday movement mechanics they are based on. When you understand this, you will be more likely to do your stretches correctly, efficiently, safely, and intelligently.

Once you understand them, you won't need to carry the stretching instructions around with you.

In Chapter 9, "Getting to Know Your Key Muscles," you will be introduced to the key muscles, their primary jobs, and the jobs they assist other muscles with. You will identify the opposing muscle for each key muscle and locate the two tendon sites. With this information you will be able to stretch in a new and knowing way. Stretching will be simple. Just follow this formula: Determine the job of the muscle you want to stretch. Then do the exact opposite motion of this job, and you will be causing the muscle to stretch.

The Formula for Stretching: Do the Exact Opposite Motion

Although this may sound simplistic, it is the most important and complete principle for stretching. Understanding it will enable you to create your own correct and safe stretching exercises, as well as allow you to see the logic behind the stretches given to you by physical therapists and doctors. Stretching intelligently—knowing exactly why you are doing what you are doing—is much more effective than stretching blindly.

To Stretch a Muscle, Contract the Opposing Muscle

Remember, the muscles work in pairs of opposites with exactly opposite jobs. Therefore, you can think of stretching this way: contracting the opposing muscle or doing the opposite job. This results in stretching the muscle. For example, if the job of the quads is to straighten the knee, contracting the opposing muscle, the hamstrings, by bending the knee will stretch the quads.

Easy Stretching

Your Back Muscles (Erector Spinae)

- Find these muscles' job: *to bend your trunk back at the hip.*
- To stretch, do the exact opposite motion: *bend your trunk forward at the hip.* (This is best done sitting on a chair.)

You can make easy stretches for all your key muscles by looking up their jobs in Chapter 9 and performing the opposite motion.

To Stretch a Muscle, Do the Exact Opposite Joint Motion

The movements at the joints can be defined in motions, such as bending forward, backward, or to the side, or rotating. These motions are the building blocks of stretches. For example, to stretch all the muscles that bend the body forward, you must bend the body backward.

Fine-Tune and Perfect the Stretch

Visualize the tendon attachments as they move farther apart (in the opposite direction from one another). Muscle movement happens when two bones connected at a joint move farther apart or closer together. When the exact locations of the two tendon sites are moved farther apart, the muscle belly is pulled out to its full length.

The multitude of excellent professional and medically correct stretching techniques available today all follow this same logic. If you apply the above principle to the stretches you get from your physical therapist, you will more easily understand what the therapist is trying to get you to do (and why!). Moreover, if you know this formula for stretching, you can stretch wherever and whenever you want, using commonsense logic to create your own stretch in response to a muscle that's asking for relief. Stretching is not a difficult, uncomfortable, or time-consuming task, and you do not need lengthy instructions, expensive gym memberships, or fancy equipment. All you need to know are the job of the muscle you want to stretch and the basic safety rules.

Many of our muscle problems stem from sitting immobile for the whole workday, performing repetitive and one-sided movements, and ignoring the signals of stress and pain that our muscles send out in response. It is not enough, nor is it always necessary, to stop the pain-generating action. In order to get relief, we must reverse the movements that are causing pain by performing the opposite action.

The Art of Stretching

Stretching is essentially an instinctual response to stiffness in our muscles and joints. It normalizes what over time has become abnormal. Unfortunately, we often ignore this instinct, remaining motionless for the entire day at our desks. In this respect, we could learn a lot from observing our pets, who have not forgotten the art of stretching.

Whenever my cat wakes up from sleeping in his favorite position, his torso bent in a circle with his head and legs curled in under it—for the spine and bones a nearly impossible position—he stretches. He elon-gates his back into an impressive arch, his legs fully straightened, and looks like he is standing on his toes. He demonstrates a perfect stretch-and-hold that includes every single muscle in his body. He holds the arched position until a little quiver goes through his body. Then he dashes for the food bowl. Even if he is starved after a long sleep curled up like that, he does not display any impatience during stretching. On the contrary, he radiates pleasure and takes his time at what seems to be an activity as important to him as breathing or eating.

When done slowly and with mental focus, stretching can be your most energizing activity because of the increased blood circulation generated and the relaxation that follows. People who practice yoga know how this feels, and stretching should be done just as slowly and meditatively as yoga, with no jerky movements whatsoever. When you get used to stretching, you will come to see it as nature's way of making our bodies feel good, relaxed, and filled with energy. You may even find yourself addicted!

How to Stretch

There are many different theories about how to stretch. A general guide-line that most agree on, however, is that stretching should be a pleasant experience that results in permanent changes rather than sore and painful muscles. You can achieve this by:

Stretching slowly enough. Stretching slowly will avoid triggering any protective emergency reactions from the tension and length monitors of the muscle being stretched. By stretching slowly, you also treat the connec-tive tissue more gently, important, since this tissue is the first to be stretched and the most impacted by stretching. Doing this will avoid pain and soreness after stretching.

Stretching far enough. Stretching beyond your normal range of move-ment is necessary to create a lasting change in the fiber length. Otherwise, the muscle will just shrink back to its original length. If you stretch only as far as your normal movement range extends, the muscle will simply main-tain this existing length. You must, therefore, bring the stretch farther than the maintaining range, which you can feel when resistance starts in the muscle.

Holding the stretch long enough. Holding the stretch until the muscle tension releases is important because it gives the length monitors time to adapt to the new length. When you hold a stretch, you can feel the tension strongly at first and then, after a while, releasing. The length you need to hold varies with the existing tension in the muscle and the varying muscle tone of each person. There are large differences in opinion over how long it is necessary to hold a stretch, with the range varying from 30 seconds to 3 minutes! As you gain experience stretching, you will be able to sense how long you need to hold until adaptation takes place.

Repeating the stretch often enough. Doing repetitions re-teaches message processing in the tissue around and inside the fibers and prevents the muscle fibers from retreating to their original pre-stretching length. Once reeducated, the muscle will retain its new length. You can stretch as often as you feel the muscle allows it. You will build an awareness of what your muscle can tolerate. When you start up, however, take into account that there is a delayed reaction in the fibers to new, unaccustomed stretching or exercising (exercise soreness). It takes a couple of days before you feel the soreness effect. Therefore, starting gently until you've come to know your muscle is the best approach to take; then add more.

Active and Passive Stretching

There are two ways to stretch:

If you bend backward in order to stretch the muscles that bend the body forward, this is an *active* stretch because you actively contract some muscles to stretch others.

Simple Stretches

Active Stretch (Calf Muscles)

- While standing, actively bend your foot and toes toward your shinbone.
- Feel the stretch in the back of your lower leg (calf).

Passive Stretch (Calf Muscles)

- Position your body on the step of a staircase.
- Scoot out so only the balls of your toes are on the step (make sure you hold onto something).
- Let the weight of your body lower your heels.
- Feel the stretch in the back of your lower legs (calves).

If you position your body, as in hanging from a bar to stretch your sides, or if you pull on a joint with your hands, this is a *passive* stretch because forces other than your own opposing muscle contraction now stretch the muscle.

These two ways of stretching are different. An active stretch is just as effective as a passive stretch, except that you activate more length and tension monitor messages when you stretch. This can be good or bad depending on the condition of the muscles you are working. Sometimes it is beneficial to be very gentle with the messaging system.

If the opposing muscle is weak, you may not be able to contract it far enough to stretch the main muscle fully. Therefore, doing a passive stretch is often a better alternative because it does not depend on the strength or weakness of the opposing muscle. By stretching passively, you can usually stretch farther and get a deeper pull by putting more pressure on the muscle.

When Will I See Results?

The time it takes to change the length of muscle fibers varies depending on how tight the muscle was to begin with. Your muscles will start feeling better soon after you start stretching. The long-term relief effect, however, appears over time. Give the fibers at least six weeks before you expect a change. When you have established a habit of stretching your muscles when they feel tight, the changes will occur without you noticing.

How to Use Chapter 12, "Stretching Your Key Muscles"

The purpose of this chapter, which provides you with stretches for individual muscles, is not to tell you how to do these but to remind you that you, like my cat, know how to stretch instinctively. By doing these stretches, you will repeatedly see the logic of the muscular system demonstrated. Check these stretches with any other stretch instructions available to you, and in the end you should have reclaimed confidence in your own ability to do what is good for your muscles without asking anyone for permission.

Before You Stretch.   Always test for tightness by doing a very slow stretch, focusing on how the muscle feels. Checking your muscle this way before you start stretching will help you determine how far you can push it during the stretch. Its purpose is to gather information about your muscle's condition so you can stretch most effectively and safely, and so that you can monitor your progress as the muscle lengthens. Doing a very slow-motion stretch first while intently listening to the signals coming from the muscle will help tune you into that particular muscle.

Warming Up.   If we had to spend a lot of time warming up before every stretch, we might never have time to stretch at all. Our objective in this book is to show that stretching is a natural movement, just like breathing, and must be done whenever the muscles ask for it. However, if you are stretching very tight and painful muscles, you will experience a remarkable difference in the effectiveness of the stretch after a warm-up as opposed to stretching without one. Warming up means improving your blood circulation before you stretch, providing extra nutrients and relaxation for the fibers, and physically raising the body temperature during the warm-up. Some good warm-ups include:

1. Walking briskly. This is the best warm-up because it gets the blood rushing through the whole body.
2. Rubbing the tendon sites and the muscle belly across the fibers. This is a great way to stimulate the circulation of messages and nutrients (as in rubbing sideways across the forearm, not along it).
3. Contracting the muscle you want to stretch tightly, holding, and then releasing. This relaxes the muscle and makes it ready for the stretch.

Starting Position.   This is a safety precaution that applies not only to stretching but to normal movements during the day as well. If you become familiar with this aligned and relaxed position, you will feel more comfortable and be more protected from injury during daily activities and stretching or strengthening exercises. The proper starting position with your body properly aligned, is described in Chapter 4.

The Stretch.   Breathe in deeply and bear the job of the muscle in mind. Stretch slowly *upon exhaling* while you visualize the location of the muscle and the two tendon sites. (It can help to review the location in Chapter 9.) Stretch as far as the muscle goes and hold. Feel the muscle tighten as the length monitors try to adjust the length back to where it was before. Then feel the muscle release as the length monitors accept that a change is indeed going to happen and adapt to it.

Ending the Stretch.   It is always a good idea to go back and check if you have lost the aligned, relaxed posture you started with. Is your tailbone still tucked under, do you still have a curve in your lower back, is your chest lifted, and is your chin tucked in just a little bit? If not, resume this safe position.

Repeating the Stretch.   Do this until you feel that the muscle is not tightening when you stretch it. As you gain experience with your muscles and practice stretching, you will develop a sensitivity to exactly when the muscle has had enough.

Overstretching

Although we have to push the tissue and muscle beyond normal range to cause a change, this does not mean we should ignore the signals our muscles send us. If you push too far too fast, you may feel the muscle pulling back strongly. You can help to avoid sending it into a spasm, which can be uncomfortable for days, by immediately bringing the muscle that is stretched into a full contraction and holding it there. This relaxes the muscle and can reverse, or reset, tension and length monitors. Other signals that the muscle will send to let you know you've gone too far are sharp pain or dull tiredness in the exact location that you were stretching. If you experience this during your stretch, stop immediately and let the muscle recover.

Remember

- Always start from and return to the safe starting position to get the best stretch.
- Always stretch slowly upon exhaling.
- Keep your mental focus on where the muscle is located.
- Stretch as far as the muscle allows and then a little more—only a stretch beyond daily range will cause change in length.
- Hold the stretch as you breathe, until you feel the muscle release.
- Repeat the stretch until the muscle has no more to give.
- Remember that the opposing muscle has been contracted during the stretch and therefore can use a stretch also.

Also remember to take into account the monitors inside the muscle itself, which constantly react and respond to any change in your muscle.

Automatic Monitoring of Your Muslces

Length Adjustments

Whenever you move, the length of the muscle fibers changes. In special situations, the length increases a lot, sometimes too fast, placing the fibers at risk of rupturing. To protect and adjust, length monitors (muscle spindle system) are spread around the muscle fibers. These report changes in length of the fibers to the central nervous system.

You can experience these monitors working when:

• You stretch too fast and too vigorously. Immediately, the muscle fibers contract and shorten as much as needed to restore the normal length (the stretch reflex). You can feel the muscle protesting for a little while before it releases. Stretching slowly is a way of giving the monitoring system time to adapt.

• The doctor taps on your knee and your lower leg moves. The length monitors think your thigh muscles (the tendons of these muscles run over the kneecap) are being stretched too fast. The tapping stretches the tendons so they contract, which straightens your leg involuntarily.

• Any time you move. Movement happens evenly and smoothly due to constant monitoring and adjusting. For example, the opposing mover relaxes when the primary mover contracts because of the length monitors.

Tension Adjustments in the Muscle Fibers

Whenever a muscle contracts or stretches, tension increases inside the muscle fibers. In unusual situations, the tension increases intensely and suddenly, placing tendon and fibers at risk of rupturing. To protect and adjust, tension monitors (Golgi tendon organs) are located right where the sac surrounding the muscle fibers becomes the tendon. They report changes in tension in the muscle fibers to the central nervous system.

You can experience these monitors working when:

• You lift a weight that demands a sudden burst of contraction, more than your fibers can handle. The contracted muscle relaxes immediately as much as needed for the situation. You may lose power and instantly drop your object. The tension was automatically and completely released to spare your tendon from rupturing.

• Your therapist deliberately applies sustained pressure to a muscle or tendon. The muscle can feel like new afterwards.

• Anytime you move. Muscle tension remains adequate for normal movement due to this constant monitoring.

CHAPTER 7

What Is Strengthening?

Have you ever been told you were slouching and needed to straighten your back? And did you try, only to sink back into a slouched position the moment you stopped thinking about your posture? After many attempts to correct your alignment, did you start worrying that there was something wrong with the bones in your back and neck? If you did, you are in good company. A lack of upper back and neck strength is one of the most common muscle dysfunctions today. It develops for very logical reasons. As we evolved, we were not meant to sit still, bending over schoolwork, office desks, or other manual work.

We can see the original intention for human movement reflected in the way the strength in our muscles is proportioned. Some muscles are stronger and some are weaker, depending on where they are in the body and what jobs they do. Those that work against gravity a lot, for example, the lower back muscles, are very strong. They need to be strong because they balance the body, resist when gravity pulls the body down and forward (so we do not fall flat on our face each time we bend a little), and pull the body back up from a bent-over position. The upper body spine, however, does not have much forward-bending range, so there was no need for the upper back muscles to be very strong.

Had we been meant to sit bent over a desk, we would have strong upper back and lower neck muscles. Yet we are created with strong lower back and leg muscles, and with weaker neck and upper back muscles, a perfectly functional design for a human wanderer who moves with head lifted and body in a predominantly upright position. For this, the upper back muscles are perfectly adequate. When we disregard this intention for movement, sitting immobile all day with a bent upper body, we change our body's situation. Already weak muscles weaken further, as a result of being held in a lengthened position. Anyone who works with muscular pain knows that even a slight change in posture can cause large changes in the health and pain level of the muscles, for better and for worse. When we look for answers to why there is such an increase in muscle pain today, it makes sense to look first at what we have changed in the way we use our bodies. Then, to avoid pain and muscle dysfunction, we can make up for the changes we have made to our movement patterns and posture.

Of course, you can't stop working at your desk. However, you can start improving your muscle condition while seated at your desk. All that is really needed is to substitute simple and adequate muscle contractions in the exact locations where weakness has developed. And once you know the logical and simple principles for strengthening a muscle, you can do this yourself whenever you need to.

The Formula for Strengthening

To strengthen a muscle, let it do its job repeatedly against resistance. For example, to bring strength back to your weakened neck and upper back muscles, and to strengthen them a little further to meet the demands of a bent-forward posture, you must not only use these muscles, but also make them work harder than normal. Merely standing in an upright position and bending backward—this muscle's job—does not cut it, because it does not provide enough resistance for the muscles to work against. But you can add resistance, for example, using gravity. If you lie on your stomach on a bed and lift your neck and head, you are providing resistance. Don't start with a full workout program, because these muscles are often both weakened and overly tense. Therefore, it is good to start with small movements and observe how the muscles contract. This helps you know when to add more power to the contractions.

How do you know that you are strengthening the right muscles? The benefit of knowing the jobs and exact locations of your muscles is that this way you can isolate a muscle, which means you will know when and how to limit a contraction to the exact muscle you want to work on. This reduces the use of unrelated muscles because all strengthening activity is happening exactly where you want it. When you look at the illustration of the neck muscles in Chapter 9, you will see that the area they cover lies right between the shoulders and moves upward. Therefore, you can scoot forward on the bed so that the area between the shoulders is on the edge while your head/neck is hanging over the edge. Now when you lift your neck backward and up, you make these precise muscles work. To isolate the upper back muscles, scoot forward a little more so the shoulders and upper back also hang over the edge. Now when you lift your chest and shoulders back up as far as they go, you are strengthening exactly those muscles that need help so desperately. Doing this exercise according to the principles of increasing muscle strength (see below) will give your upper back the strength it needs.

What Is Needed to Increase Strength?

As with stretching, there are many theories about how best to strengthen muscles, but most experts agree on certain basic elements. A muscle must be used (contracted), and it must be pushed beyond the normal daily level of usage. There is an important difference, however, between stretching and strengthening. Stretching a painful muscle contributes to its healing, while strengthening a painful muscle can add to its problem. Therefore, if a muscle is painful when you do strengthening exercises, you should stop. The fibers need to heal before they are able to handle the extra load of strengthening.

During strengthening work you must:

1. Contract the muscle as far as it goes. Each time, lift or bend as far as you can, to the full available pain-free range of motion.
2. Repeat the movement enough times. You should do two or three sets of from 3 to 10 repetitions, depending on the weight used and the kind of muscle contraction used (see below). Often you will have to determine the ideal number of repetitions for your body based on how your muscles feel and respond.
3. Strengthen the muscles often enough. A set of repetitions three times a week is the minimum needed for strengthening to succeed.

Even a single strengthening contraction does a ton of good for your muscle. The tissue between the fibers is pushed and shoved, which helps to prevent it from adhering, or gluing together. Blood flow gets a jump start, the message communication system is awakened, and the fibers get exercised. All of this contributes to making you feel better for much the same reasons that stretching does.

There are several ways to work a muscle. Therefore, you can choose to use one strengthening technique, or you can add complexity step-by-step as you go. Here are some strengthening techniques:

1. Tense the muscle by contracting it as tightly as you can without moving your body (isometric contraction: *iso* = same, *metro* = length). This is a very good exercise to help you retain or regain muscle strength if

you are sick in bed and cannot move around. In fact, it is also great to do while you are sitting still at work during the day.

2. Contract the muscle by letting the muscle do its job (concentric contraction.) This is how you use the muscles in normal daily movement, but a muscle will strengthen only if you contract it all the way to full range!

STRENGTHEN YOUR STOMACH MUSCLES THE EASY WAY

It is important for your back that you have strong abdominal muscles. Using isometric contraction, you can strengthen them anytime and anywhere. Just tense your stomach muscles—hold for a couple of seconds and let go slowly, not like a punctured balloon. Repeat this often during the day, and slowly your stomach muscles will strengthen.

3. Add resistance. Make the muscle work harder by using gravity or weights for resistance (concentric contraction).

4. Contract and stretch at the same time. Make the muscle work even harder by contracting it as it is being stretched (eccentric contraction). This generates even more strength because the muscle has to do several things at the same time. For example, when you lie on the floor on your back with your head lifted toward your chest and then lower your head very slowly down to the floor, the front neck muscles are being stretched (lengthened as the head is lowered) at the same time as they contract (to hold back the head so it does not fall to the floor). Because the fibers slowly lengthen while holding, doubled fiber work occurs. You will have noticed this if you have done knee-bending exercises. The front of your thighs, the quads, gets heavily taxed. When you bend your knee, lowering your body, these muscles contract, holding the weight of your body to prevent it from falling to the floor, while at the same time they are being slowly stretched. You can end up with more soreness after strengthening this way. This is something to be aware of, as overdoing can punish you.

Contract and Stretch at the Same Time

Eccentric contraction is the most effective workout for your muscles. To do it, hold a weight in your hand with your elbow bent to 90 degrees, then slowly lower the weight toward the floor.

The front upper arm muscles must contract all the time to prevent the weight from dropping and are being stretched at the same time as you lower the weight.

Your daily activities are always a combination of these different ways of using the muscles. When you deliberately want to strengthen a muscle, however, it is helpful to know that you have options. You may need to work in different ways, depending on your situation.

Muscle Changes

When we strengthen our muscles, the muscle fibers themselves change. There are actual physical changes occurring. Two things happen: the diameter of the fibers increases (hypertrophy) and the number of fibers are thought to increase (hyperplasia). There is also a definite change in the way the fibers react. They kick in faster, and more fibers are activated in response to the messages from the central nervous system. Last, and most important for people with muscle pain, the number of blood vessels (capillaries) increases radically, bringing more blood to the muscle.

Unfortunately, we also have to contend with the other side of the coin, which is that the exact reversal of these good effects takes place when we do not strengthen our muscles. Strength does not remain in the muscles when you do not use them. Thus, immobility reduces the strength. The fibers of the muscles that are kept immobile diminish in size and number. It is not only during illness that muscle fibers weaken quickly. It happens anytime a muscle isn't being used. This is what the saying "Use it or lose it!" means.

To keep muscles from weakening and to maintain their strength, you only need to move normally and make up for time spent sitting still by adding an equal amount of motion. However, if you want to benefit from the improvements in muscle health that result from strengthening, you must go beyond daily motion. You must make the muscle work until it tires.

This book focuses on improving endurance strength. The reason for this is that during the use of low-level resistance and many repetitions (as opposed to lifting heavy weights), the first thing that happens is crucial to relieving muscle pain and increasing health: the number of blood vessels (capillaries) inside the muscle increases rapidly. They have been found to increase by as much as 20 percent after only eight weeks of training and following an intense exercise program. The increase in blood vessels does not occur in as dramatic a fashion with power-training methods.

What this means is that to achieve normal, healthy, pain-free muscles, you do not have to become a weightlifting expert. Rather than lifting heavy weights, you can strengthen your muscles easily just by using enough resistance and repetitions to exceed your normal daily usage.

How Strong Is Strong Enough?

A child does not have very strong muscles, but most likely the balance between the child's muscles is healthy. This is all we are trying for—an adequate strength for normal function and balance between the muscles in the group. Therefore, the strength of a muscle is not an entity that should be measured alone, but rather in relation to the other muscles in the group it belongs to.

Balance

Most people with weak upper back muscles have too strong or tight front-of-the-shoulder muscles (pectorals). These are the opposing muscles to the upper back muscles. Because the main mover and the opposing muscle work in synchronicity, what affects one also affects the other. Tight pectoralis muscles make it even harder for the back muscles to do their job. We now have a second explanation for why we slouch, and a second task: to stretch out and release the pectoralis muscles so they no longer prevent the upper back muscles from doing their job. Stretching releases tightness and hypercontraction.

Strength inequality between muscles with opposing functions is one of the first things to look at before treating muscle pain conditions. Good strength training programs always make sure that when you increase the strength of one muscle, you also increase the strength of the opposing muscle to avoid imbalance.

Strength is important, not because a muscle necessarily has to be strong to be pain-free, but rather because a muscle must have adequate and balanced strength.

How to Use Chapter 13, "Strengthening Your Key Muscles"

Testing a muscle or muscle group for strength and achieving precise results is not a simple thing. At a health club, you can use electronic technical equipment that measures the power with which you pull a rope or lift a weight. Most physical therapists use manual muscle testing (providing resistance with their own hands). They evaluate your strength based on their knowledge, experience, and accepted professional standards that determine minimum strength levels for a functional muscle. If you have a wide variety of weights at your disposal, you can test for the maximum amount of weight you are able to lift through the range of motion for one repetition. With this same method, you can measure your endurance and see how many repetitions of a certain motion you can carry out through the full range.

Make Your Own Weights

- Use a long sock.
- Put two cans in the sock; these can be one-pound or two-pound cans, depending on your need.
- Before you tie off the end, insert a stick into the length of your homemade weight; this makes it easier to hold. Leave a space for your hand between the two cans. You can use a ruler, a wooden stick, or any solid bar you have available.

What we really want to know is not if our muscles are weak or strong, but rather if they have the symptoms of change away from what is healthy. We need to know if the muscle has enough strength in relation to its group. We are not looking for weak muscles, but for weakened muscles.

The test is based on a method that many physical therapists use to measure the minimum strength for a functional muscle.

Testing

Always test your muscles for symptoms before you strengthen. Then do one strengthening exercise slowly, listening to and feeling how the muscle works. Put the muscle under the microscope of your attention, paying special note to any sensation deviating from an even and smooth contraction. There should be no pain, no shaking, no tremor, and no loss of power. Although the exercises presented in this book normally do not cause sore muscles, it is still a good idea to stretch the muscle slowly and thoroughly several times before you start strengthening.

Strengthening

Remember: Even if you do not feel strong enough to tackle the minimum repetitions and weights, it is beneficial to do even a single strengthening exercise. Bear in mind that the number of repetitions suggested in Chapter 13 is the minimum required for strengthening to occur. You will not be able to strengthen your muscles if the level is too low, so experiment and adapt the exercises to what feels right. You may need to add more repetitions and weight.

After Strengthening

Stretching again afterward relieves the muscle fibers of the tension created during the workout and helps prevent soreness.

> ### Remember:
> Whenever you strengthen the primary muscle, always strengthen the opposing muscle as well.
>
> When you strengthen the primary muscle, you also improve the strength in the assisting muscles for that action.

Listen to your muscles during and after exercising! If you experience severe exhaustion or strain in a muscle, you may need to reduce weight, repetitions, or both.

CHAPTER 8

Step By Step Toward Relief

This chapter shows you how to move from knowing that you hurt in a particular spot to taking concrete and effective steps toward identifying, treating, and relieving the painful muscle or muscle group that might be involved.

First we will guide you to find the right muscle, or muscles, to work on, and then we will take you, step by step, through the process of learning to relieve them of tension and pain. At the end of this chapter, you'll find a couple of examples of how to use this approach.

To start: Point to the part of your body that hurts. You can let the step-by-step guide help you do the rest.

Step 1: Find Your Key Muscle

Your first task is to find the name of the key muscle that is located in the spot you are pointing to, using the Quick Reference at the back of the book.

Determine which part of your body this spot is located in (such as the arm, thigh, lower leg, hip, or trunk). Once that's accomplished, turn to the Quick Reference in the back of the book. Look through the headings (shoulder, knee, etc.). Each section provides more detailed locations to choose from, such as the front, back, side, outside, or inside of the body part involved.

Here you will find one or more key muscle names listed. Now that you know the name of your key muscle, it is time to move to Step 2 to learn about this muscle's characteristics. If there is more than one muscle listed, follow the instructions in Steps 2 and 3 for each one. By testing them, you will soon realize which of these is your key muscle, the muscle most in need of healing.

Step 2: Get to Know Your Key Muscle

This step will help you to collect information about your key muscle. Read about it in Chapter 9. This chapter tells you about the muscle's job, its location, and its typical traits. Locate the tendons, feel the muscle move as it contracts or stretches, and also read about the group of muscles it works closely with.

Now it's time to proceed to Step 3.

Step 3. Test Your Key Muscle

Turn to Chapter 11, which provides you with a range of motion test to carry out, and to the end of Chapter 10, which explains how to use the testing chapter. Test the range of motion of your key muscle to see if it is tighter than it should be. For example, if the job of your key muscle is to bend your neck forward, turn to the section called "Neck Tests" and then turn to "Bending Forward." Follow the instructions and take notes as you test the condition of your key muscle.

Do a slow stretch test. The index will refer you to stretches for your key muscle. Pay attention to the sensations in your body. Does it feel tight or painful to perform the stretch?

Test the level of pain in your key muscle. Gently press on and around each tendon site, searching for areas that are tender or sore. Carefully rub along the belly of the muscle, from one tendon to the other, to see if you find tender and sore or swollen and warm areas.

Test the strength of your key muscle. If the muscle is not too painful, do a careful, gentle strengthening exercise. The index will refer you to strengthening exercises for your key muscle. This means that you contract the muscle and observe how it works.

Step 4: Start the Healing Process

Now it's time to try out a variety of techniques to stimulate the circulation, massage, soothe, calm, relax, and heal your muscle. To begin, turn to Chapter 5. Do the exercises listed in the activity boxes in this section as they relate to your key muscle.

To help relax muscles that will not relax by themselves, use the techniques in Chapter 5., using the activity boxes.

Alternating use of ice and hot packs can effectively reduce swelling and relieve pain. Chapter 5 tells you how to make your own ice and hot packs as well as how to use them.

When the muscle starts to heal as you provide circulation aid and stretching, strengthening completes the healing process.

Step 5: Stretch and Strengthen Your Key Muscle

Before you start doing the stretches, turn to Chapter 4, which describes the safe aligned starting position for any activity. Now turn to Chapter 6, which describes how to do the stretches, and then to Chapter 12, which provides the stretches. Slowly stretch your muscle. The stretch paragraph you use will give you the name of your key muscle's opposing muscle; stretch this muscle, too.

Chapter 6, "What Is Stretching?" explains the stretching principle, which is based on the job the muscle has.

Repeat the same routine for strengthening. Read Chapter 7, "What Is Strengthening?," to learn what it takes to strengthen muscle fibers, and then turn to Chapter 13, which provides the strengthening exercises.

Step 6: Be Mindful of Your Muscles during the Day

Armed with the information about your key muscle, turn to the Chapter 4 section, "Analyze Your Daily Activities." You need to determine if you use your key muscle repetitively during the course of the day or if you tend to hold it immobile in one position. With this awareness, you can now pay attention to your key muscle during the day, relieve your pain, and stretch the muscle whenever you feel the need. You are no longer compounding the pain, but taking steps to prevent it in the future.

Step 7: See the Bigger Picture of Your Pain

A muscle does not work alone. Turn to the key muscle section in Chapter 9 and look for the group your muscle works in. Find the name of the muscle that opposes the work of your key muscle. This muscle has a major influence on your key muscle. Repeat the same steps with this opposing muscle that you took for your key muscle.

Next, locate and read about the muscles that assist your key muscles. You'll find these, too, in Chapter 9. Repeat the same steps with each of these.

Read Chapter 4, which explains how muscles work together in pairs and groups, for more information. Also read the section that explains how to align your body to take the burden off your pained muscle(s).

How Often, How Much, and for How Long Should You Work Your Muscles?

The relief from pain can be almost immediate when you start supplying your muscle with increased blood flow and exercise, or it can take time, depending on how much and how long it has been hurting.

When you start massaging, stretching, and exercising, you necessarily stir things up. This is good for your tissue and muscles. Still, your muscles may react by becoming somewhat sore and tender, due, among other things, to an increase in the production of waste products due to micro-trauma at first from the uncustomary treatment. (Read Chapter 2 for more information about the waste products and pain sensation.)

Therefore, if you experience some worsening in the beginning, this is often a part of the healing process. As you work, it is essential to develop sensitivity to your muscles and tissues so you can distinguish between good and bad pain. Also see Chapter 2 about the difference between acute and chronic pain. As a rule of thumb, if you experience symptoms that seem like acute pain—sharp, new, unaccustomed pain—stop your relief work, rest, and consult a doctor. Pain that is more of the same, even if it increases, is a natural part of the healing process and will diminish the more you work to repair your muscle. How often to stretch is up to how you feel, but a minimum of two to three stretching routines per day to begin with, doing at least five repetitions, is recommended; then soon progress to four to five routines per day.

Persistent, gentle, but firm treatment over time brings results. Tissue, fibers, and nerve input need time to change. After six to eight weeks of stretching, you may feel that your range has changed for the better. The same is true for strengthening. Here are some examples of muscle pain and the appropriate course of action for each.

Example 1

You experience frequent pain and soreness in the back of your thigh, close to your buttocks. You know the source of your pain is somewhere in this vicinity—after all, that's where it hurts! But you're not sure just which muscles are involved. To find out, you decide to use the Quick Reference.

Step 1. Find Your Key Muscle.   To help get a better sense of exactly where the pain begins and ends, you reach behind your thigh and touch this area. In the Quick Reference you find the heading "Thigh" reading further, you find the subsection that covers the back of the thigh. Eureka! You discover that the muscles operating here are the hamstrings.

Step 2. Get to Know Your Key Muscle.   You have pinpointed the hamstring muscles as the source of your problem. Looking them up in Chapter 9, you learn that the hamstrings' job is to bend the knee, you learn that these muscles attach to the lowest part of the hipbone in the buttocks and also to the outsides of the knee in the back.

Step 3. Test Your Key Muscle.   Your next step is to determine the extent of your problem by testing your key muscle. You turn to the section of Chapter 11 called "Bending the Knee" and test the range of motion of your hamstrings. You discover that they are very tight and painful to stretch. Feeling along the muscle belly, moving from one tendon to the other, you realize that all the tendon sites are sore and that the muscle belly feels almost rock hard and sore also. You determine that your hamstring muscles are just too sore to work with. Even a slow stretch hurts badly. You decide not to do any strengthening exercise at this stage.

Step 4. Start the Healing Process.   Following the instructions and suggestions in Chapter 5, you carefully treat your hamstrings by massaging tendon sites and the muscle belly always ending with a gentle stretch. As you persist over several days, you begin to find that the pain is subsiding.

Step 5. Stretch and Strengthen Your Key Muscle.   Your next step is to stretch and strengthen, so you turn to Chapter 12. There you find stretches under the "Knee" heading ("Bending the Knee") and learn to gently stretch your hamstrings, using no sudden movements. After some time, you find that the pain has diminished and it is time to start strengthening. So you turn to Chapter 13 again and look in the "Knee" section under "Bending the Knee." You learn how to very gently strengthen your hamstrings.

Step 6. Be Mindful of Your Muscles during the Day.   You realize that your desk job requires you to sit on your hamstrings all day. Using Chapter 5, you teach yourself how to provide blood flow to these muscles during the day. You read Chapter 4 and learn to revise your workday routine, taking frequent short breaks to get up and gently stretch these muscles.

Step 7: See the Bigger Picture of Your Pain.   You are well enough to start thinking preventively. You return to Chapter 9 and look up the hamstrings muscle group, and discover that the quads are the opposing muscles to the hamstrings. You repeat the steps you took to heal your key muscles for your quads. Finally, you return to Chapter 9 and look up the muscles that assist the hamstrings to bend the knees. You treat these also.

Example 2

The painful spot is in the back of your upper arm.

Step 1. Find Your Key Muscle. To get a clear idea of exactly where the painful area is, you reach around and touch the back of your upper arm.

You turn to Appendix 1, the Quick Reference, where you get the key muscles, the triceps and deltoid posterior. Having located and checked out the illustrations of both muscles in Chapter 9, you decide to start with the triceps because this muscle seems to be the one located closest to where the pain is.

Step 2. Get to Know Your Key Muscle. Under "Typical Traits," you read that the back and outside of your upper arm often get sore thanks to a stressed triceps muscle. That rings a bell. Now you know you are on the right track. You also read that it is common for people who work with their hands extended in front of their bodies to have sore triceps. You happen to do that. Now you are even closer to verifying that this might indeed be the muscle causing your pain. You follow the instructions to find the tendons and muscle belly.

(Note that problems with the rotary cuff muscles often show up as pain in the back of the upper arm, so this might need to be checked out. They are not included in this book.)

Step 3. Test Your Key Muscle. You now want to determine the extent of the problem. Since the job of the triceps is to straighten your arm at the elbow, you go to Chapter 11 under the heading "Elbow Tests" and perform the range of motion test for your triceps. Your range is normal, but the muscle is painful. You read the "Interpreting Your Results" section in Chapter 10, which explains that a muscle can be weakened and painful even if it the range is normal, especially if gravity helps do the muscle's job. You notice that gravity helps straighten your arm, so your triceps never get much strengthening during normal activities, and are probably weak and need strengthening.

When you reach under to find the tendon on the shoulder blade close to the armpit and then press in deep, it hurts. Your next move is to find the other tendons. This muscle ends on the elbow, on a tendon shared by the three parts of the muscle. This tendon is not as sore as the one on the shoulder blade. Checking the description in the text as you go, you find the muscle belly lying between the two tendons. Yes, here is the pain you first felt. Rubbing the muscle belly hurts a little bit, but the most intense pain is on the shoulder blade. You have now expanded your pain information to include a connection between the muscle in the back of your upper arm and the newly discovered sore spot on your shoulder blade.

Step 4. Start the Healing Process.   Next, you turn to Chapter 5 and learn how and where to perform tendon and muscle belly massage. This hurts while you do it, but it's a good kind of pain—you feel you're getting somewhere at last. You end the treatment with a slow triceps stretch.

Step 5. Stretch and Strengthen Your Key Muscle.   Chapter 9 refers you to the triceps stretch in Chapter 12. You start stretching this muscle at least five times during your day. After a while, you feel a need to stretch even more often. You read Chapter 6, "What Is Stretching?" and learn more about how to stretch anytime, anywhere. You decide it is too sore to strengthen at this point, and therefore you wait a couple of weeks before you start gentle strengthening.

Step 6. Be Mindful of Your Muscles.   In Chapter 4, "Taking the Burden Off Your Muscles," you discover how you have been stretching your triceps for long hours by holding your arm extended in front of you with elbows bent. You now know it needs strengthening. You learn how performing the opposite motion, simply straightening your arm, helps you regain balanced usage and relieves your triceps muscle. You find yourself starting to pay attention to your triceps during the day, noticing consciously what you've been doing to it unconsciously. Intermittently, you extend your arm backward, straight and close to your body, and hold the position for a second or two. This gently strengthens the triceps and relieves it from the stress of your customary outstretched position.

Step 7. See the Bigger Picture of Your Pain.   You realize that you need to put the problem in a bigger context to lay it to rest, so you return to the key muscle section and find the muscles that interact with your triceps, starting with the opposing muscle, the biceps. You realize what a strength and usage difference there is between these two muscles; the biceps is continually strengthened through bending the arm and lifting things. Gradually, you acquire the habit of paying attention to both these muscles—massaging, stretching, and strengthening, and viewing these two muscles as a pair, each influencing the other's condition. Last, you look up and test the assisting muscles as well.

Example 3

Your painful spot is on the outside of your hip, right where the body bends when you sit.

Step 1. Find Your Key Muscle.   To better get an idea of exactly where the pain is located, you touch and press in deep. The spot is hard and bony. You determine that it is close to a joint, the hip. After checking the joint description in Chapter 10, which convinces you that it is indeed the hip joint you are looking at, you turn to the Quick Reference and look under the headings "Hip" and "Side." It lists many key muscles—gluteus maximus, gluteus medius, piriformis, and tensor fasciae latae. Don't despair. Go back to the beginning of the step-by-step guide, where you find an explanation of what to do.

Following these instructions, you learn that all these muscles have a tendon that attaches to the bone in the side of your hip/thigh that is causing you pain. This means that while all these muscles work, they pull on your sore spot.

To determine which muscle is your troublemaker, you look at the muscle jobs. Slowly and attentively, you perform the jobs of each of these muscles in turn. You notice that rotating the thigh gives rise to pain deep inside your buttocks. Hmm; the piriformis is the key muscle whose main job it is to rotate the thigh outward. It attaches to your sore spot, and it hurts to contract it. Now you've made the connection between a hurting bone and a tight, painful buttock muscle. You look at the illustration of the piriformis and find that it is located right there, deep inside your buttocks. The detective work is over; this is most likely the key muscle you need to work on.

Step 2. Get to Know Your Key Muscle.   You read all about this muscle. You know that you have a habit of crossing your left leg and placing the foot on your other knee, a practice that strongly rotates the hip outward. This contracts your piriformis continuously. You are beginning to see a reason for the pain in this muscle.

Step 3. Test Your Key Muscle.   You have already found tender sore areas on and around where the ending tendon of your key muscle is, and you know that the muscle belly is sore inside your buttocks, so you stretch, which hurts quite a lot. You decide against strengthening this muscle because it feels so tight and painful. You decide to move on to testing the range of motion.

You turn to Chapter 11, "Testing Your Key Muscles." You turn to the hip and thigh section, where you find that the motion of your muscle is "rotating the thigh outward." You follow the instructions and learn that your range is normal; however, when you test the opposite movement, rotating the thigh *inward,* your range is very limited. This is crucial information about your piriformis. You've been told already that when you do the opposite motion of the muscle's job, you stretch it. Since the range is limited when you stretch the muscle, you know it is tight and needs stretching.

Step 4. Start the Healing Process.   You are reminded that it is also painful and needs relief work, so you go to Chapter 5 and, using the techniques described, start increasing the circulation to your muscle and help it relax. You work on the part of this muscle that you can get to. Part of it is inside your buttocks.

Step 5. Stretch and Strengthen Your Key Muscle.   You already know the stretch for this muscle. You start stretching this muscle at least five times a day. This is not that hard, since simply rotating the thigh inward—the opposite motion—is a good stretch. You do this standing up, with your hands on the side and top of the thighbone, always starting in the starting position (see Chapter 4), just by turning your foot inward while you feel the rotation under your hand.

Step 6. Be Mindful of Your Muscles during the Day.   You already know what you are doing that aggravates this muscle, so you try to remember not to sit with your leg in this position, and as often as you remember, you turn your thigh inward instead of outward. Whenever you feel tightness, you stretch this muscle.

Step 7. See the Bigger Picture of Your Pain.   In Chapter 9, you look up the opposing and assisting muscles. You build stretching these into your daily routine, too.

Remember, there are far more muscles in the body than the 36 discussed in this book, and your pain might stem from some of them. The key muscles in this book, however, are the main movers of your main joints, so it is very likely that one or more of these 36 is the culprit.

There is one exception: The biceps muscle, which bends your arm. This is a muscle most people already know. That it is not included among the key muscles does not mean it isn't a frequent troublemaker. Now that you know what to look for—its job, its location, and its tendon attachments—we recommend that you find books on muscles in the bookstore and get to know it before it causes you pain.

Part Two

CHAPTER 9

Getting to Know
Your Key Muscles

This chapter is the backbone of the book: a detailed introduction to 36 key muscles in your body, their main functions (jobs), and the task each performs at a joint, such as bending or straightening, for example, your knee. To locate a muscle in the body is not a mysterious matter that should only be attempted by a therapist. Learn how to find each muscle and the exact sites at which it attaches to the bone, how to feel the muscle move while it is contracting or stretching, and the typical traits of that muscle. In addition, you'll discover which muscles work closely with each key muscle, the muscle group it belongs to that has a strong impact on its health and function. With this information, you can begin the healing process.

You will find that each of the 36 key muscle descriptions in this chapter are organized the same way:

"Bony Landmarks." Each joint section starts with an explanation of bony landmarks. This is because finding the muscle attachment sites is much easier when you have found and recognized in advance the feel of the many bumps and bones that the muscles attach to. Bony landmarks will be in quotation marks so that you can more easily recognize these in the text.

"Job." Under this heading you will find listed the different jobs of the muscle, starting with its primary job and then its assisting jobs. When you see "(both muscles working)" under the job description, this means that the pair of muscles on either side of the spine, which are exact copies of each other, both participate in the movement described. Otherwise, you can assume that only one muscle is involved in the movement.

"How to Find It." This section guides you to exactly where the muscle itself and its two tendons are located. To differ between these two sites, we say that a muscle begins on one bone and ends on another. If a muscle has several parts, each part will have a separate beginning or ending tendon and share the other tendon. A shared tendon, the common tendon, is a great place to massage to relieve pain and tension, since it carries a heavier load. You will find that a large part of the muscle description is devoted to locating tendon sites. This will help you understand the dynamics of your stretches as well as how to heal and prevent tendinitis.

"Typical Traits." Here you'll find some characteristics that will help you recognize your key muscle, such as how and when it is most likely to get hurt, accompanied by a couple of improvement tips for this particular muscle. Some muscles tend to need strengthening to improve their condition, while others are most likely to need stretching. The section ends with the potential benefits of treating this particular muscle.

"Group." This section lists other muscles that are affected if the key muscle is tight or painful, namely, the muscles that work closely with your key muscle. This includes the muscle whose function is to perform the opposite job of your key muscle, the opposing muscle, and the muscle(s) that assist your key muscle with that function, the opposing muscle and the assisting muscles.

Muscles of the Neck

Bony Landmarks for Locating Muscles that Move the Head and Neck

How to Find Them

Skull.   This refers to the bony surface of the head bone, stretching from ear to ear.

Vertebrae of the neck.   These are the bones along the upper spine, C1 through C7. The "C" stands for "cervical" (neck), and the numbers refer to the individual vertebrae that feel like bumps under the skin. They are numbered sequentially from the top down, starting with C1. The last and biggest neck vertebra (C7) sticks out the most.

Breastbone (sternum).   This narrow, flat, vertical bone extends down the chest; this is where the ribs attach.

Collarbone (clavicle).   What we call the collarbone are the two horizontal bones on top of the chest that extend in opposite directions from the breastbone, to within about an inch of the tip of the shoulder joint.

Bending Forward (Flexion) Muscle

The two-part sternocleidomastoid (SCM) muscle moves and protects the head and the neck. The long name refers to the three bones this muscle attaches to: the "breastbone" (*sterno*—sternum), the "collarbone" (*cleido*—clavicle), and the "skull" (*mastoid*—mastoid process) right behind the ears.

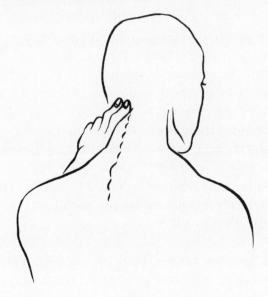

Neck

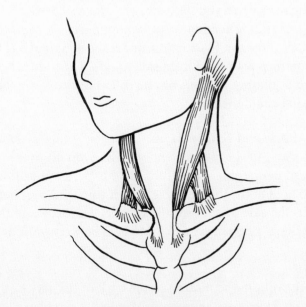

Sternocleidomastoid

Job

Bends the head forward and down to the chest (flexion) (both muscles working)

Also:

Rotates the head to the opposite side (rotation)
Helps to bend the neck to the same side, toward the muscle (lateral flexion)
Resists when the head is pulled backward forcefully, as in whiplash
Helps to lift the rib cage during forced breathing

How to Find It

To find the first beginning tendon, place your fingers on top of the breastbone where the collarbones meet in front. As you bend your head backward, press on the bone in the indentation; you will sense the tendon as a slightly squishy band being pulled under the skin. When you rotate your head from side to side, this tendon and muscle stand out very prominently from the breastbone and protrude from the front of your neck. To find the other beginning tendon, place your fingers on your collarbone, positioned about one and a half inches from where the collarbones meet, toward the shoulder. Push in on the upper edge of the bone and feel how the tendon tightens when you tilt your head and neck back.

To find the ending tendon, place your fingers on the skull directly behind and below the ear. Press in just under the bone and feel the tendon moving as you turn your head from side to side. The muscle belly extends from the two beginning tendons on the collarbone to share the common ending tendon behind the ear.

To Feel the Muscle and Tendon Move: Place your fingers about one and a half inches above the beginning tendons while you tilt your head back or turn your head to one side, away from the muscle, as far as it will go. You can also grab hold of the thick muscle belly if you bend your head forward and a little to the side away from the muscle. The belly and the tendons stand out, making it easy for you to grab them between your fingers.

Typical Traits

It is natural to point to the muscles at the back of the neck as the cause of most neck pain. However, the front SCM muscles can play a large part in neck pain as well. Keeping your neck bent forward while working at a desk for extended periods of time eventually compacts and shortens these muscles. The SCM muscles react to abuse by becoming tight, short, and weak.

Improvement Tip: Adjust your head and neck position, and provide a tension-releasing stretch by lifting your chin often and tilting the head backward and to the sides. Provide circulation aid, stretching, and gentle strengthening.

Payoff: Tight SCM muscles and headaches often go hand in hand. Stretching and strengthening exercises can help restore a balanced head and neck position, giving relief to the muscles at the back of the neck, and thus greatly reducing headaches.

Group

Opposing Muscle: In bending forward, the two splenii muscles, which bend the head and neck backward.

Assisting Muscles: In bending forward, both sides of the scalene muscles. For rotating the head to the opposite side, the front part of the scalenes on the opposite side. In tilting the head to the same side, the scalene and splenii on the same side.

Bending Backward (Extension)

The two splenii muscles work together to bend the head and neck backward. They resemble two patches on the neck. The upper patch is the splenius capitis, and the lower patch is the splenius cervicis. Splenius means *patch,* capitis means *head* (this muscle moves the head), and cervicis means *neck* (this muscle moves the neck).

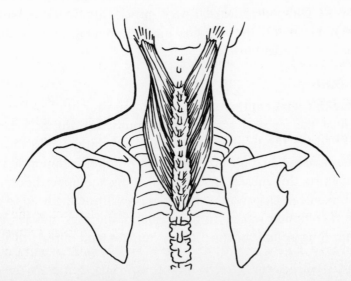

Splenius capitis and splenius cervicis

Job:

Tilts the head and neck backward (extension).

Also:

Helps to tilt the head and neck to the same side (lateral flexion).

How to Find It

Upper (splenius capitis): To find the beginning tendons, place your hands on your spine at the neck and run your fingers down the vertebrae (which will feel like bumps) starting from one inch under the skull. On the backs of the five vertebrae, C3 through C7, are the tendon attachments. The muscle belly creates a V-shaped cover on the neck and reaches up to the skull.

To find the ending tendon, place your fingers at the center of the back of your "skull," and then feel out toward your ear, about two inches from the center. You will reach a slight dent right under the bone. By pressing your fingers on and under the bone, you should be able to feel the tendon as it is being pulled when you tilt your head forward. The tendon here is often so tense that it creates a sore area (a great place to massage).

Lower (splenius cervicis): This muscle, which has the same V shape as the splenius capitis, is located on the neck right under the splenius capitis. It begins lower down on the spine and ends on the sides of the upper-neck vertebrae (C1–C3).

To Feel the Muscles Move: Place one hand on each side of the biggest neck vertebra (C7) and press in deeply while you tilt your head backward and forward. Only one other flat neck muscle, the trapezius, covers this area, so you can feel the splenius muscles moving underneath. (The trapezius is a shoulder muscle.)

Typical Traits

These muscles work continuously to maintain your head and neck position against the force of gravity, which pulls forward, backward, and sideways. Tilting the head forward while hunching over a desk keeps these muscles stretched for hours on end. Another common head position that hurts this muscle involves hunching the upper body (maybe with a sunken chest) forward, which requires lifting the head to see, for example, a computer screen. In this scenario, the neck muscles are contracted for long periods of time. These muscles tend to react to abuse by becoming weak (they are not strong to begin with) and by accumulating tension.

Improvement Tip: Adjust your upper body, head, and neck position and provide circulation aid and gentle stretching, then strengthening exercises.

Payoff: You get relief from stiffness and pain in the back of your neck and when turning your head to the side. You can also help relieve headaches.

Group
Opposing Muscle: In bending backward, both SCMs, which bend the head and neck forward.

Assisting Muscles: In bending backward, the upper trapezius (when the shoulder is fixed) and the neck part of the erector spinae. In bending to the same side, the scalene and the SCM on the same side.

Bending Sideways (Lateral Flexion)
The scalenes encompass three muscles: the scalenus anterior, medius, and posterior. They work together almost as one muscle to bend the head to the side. Scalenes means *odd, uneven, bent, crooked;* anterior means *front;* medius *middle,* and posterior, *back.*

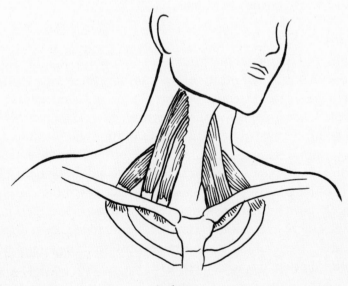

Scalenes

Job

> Tilts the head directly to the same side as the muscle (ear to shoulder movement; lateral flexion)

Also:

> Helps to bend the neck forward (cervical flexion)
> Lifts the ribs during inhalation.
> Helps to rotate the head to the opposite side

How to Find It

The beginning tendons (front, middle, and back): These muscles begin on the side of the neck vertebrae (C2–C6), so you won't be able to reach the tendons with your hands. From the neck, the muscle bellies angle out toward the shoulder.

To find the ending tendons on the ribs directly beneath the "collarbone," place your fingers on and above the "collarbone" halfway between your "breastbone" and the tip of your shoulder. Press deeply on the upper inside of the bone and feel these tendons stretch when you tilt your head to the opposite side.

To Feel the Muscles Move: Press in on the side of the neck, two inches above the "collarbone," while you tilt your head directly to one side and get the feel of these frequently tight muscles.

Typical Traits

It is thanks to the scalenes that your head does not flop to the side but is maintained in a centered position. You can hurt these muscles by tilting the head to the side for extended periods of time and overloading one side, for example, while holding the phone between ear and shoulder. (One side reacts to being contracted for long periods of time and the other to being stretched.) Also, carrying something heavy on one shoulder (such as a purse with a strap) can cause the scalenes on this side to tighten. A habit of shallow breathing keeps the scalenes shortened. When the rib cage does not fall back down fully, the scalenes are not allowed to lengthen, and soon you may be caught in a vicious cycle where it is hard to relax both the chest and the neck. These muscles are very sensitive to changes and tense up, tighten, and shorten in reaction to abuse.

Improvement Tip: Relax your shoulders and chest. Use circulation aids, including breathing exercises, and slow, gentle stretching.

Payoff: By treating your scalenes, you may experience freedom from tightness and pain that is felt on the side and at the back of the neck, as well as an increased sense of relaxation. You can also help prevent arm and wrist problems such as carpal tunnel syndrome, because when the ribs remain lifted, close to the collarbone, due to tight scalenes, this prevents the blood vessels and nerves that pass under the collarbone and over the first rib from supplying the arms and wrists (thoracic outlet syndrome). Therefore, tight neck muscles can cause pain in your arms, wrists, and fingers.

Group

Opposing Muscle: In bending to the same side, the scalene on the opposite side, which bends the head and neck to the opposite side.

Assisting Muscles: In bending to the same side, the SCM and levator scapulae on the same side. In forward bending and in lifting the ribs, the SCMs.

Muscles of the Shoulder

Bony Landmarks for Locating Muscles that Move the Shoulder

How to Find Them

Upper edge of the shoulder blade (spine of the scapula).   With one hand, reach over the shoulder and feel the bony ridge on top of the shoulder blade that extends to the "tip of the shoulder."

Tip of the shoulder joint (acromion process).   Follow the "upper edge of the shoulder blade" out to the tip of the shoulder and feel how the bone becomes bigger and meets the collarbone at the tip of the shoulder.

Upper inner corner of the shoulder blade (superior angle).   This is the upper corner closest to the spine. Reach over your shoulder and follow the "upper edge of the shoulder blade" in to where it ends about one and a half to two inches from the spine.

Inner edge of the shoulder blade.   Reach over your shoulder and position your hand on the "upper inner corner of the shoulder blade." Try to feel the inner edge of the shoulder blade as it runs down the midback parallel with your spine.

Outer edge of the shoulder blade.   Reach under your armpit and find your shoulder blade. The outer edge is close to your side. To help you locate and feel the outer edge of the blade, move your arm, which also moves the shoulder blade.

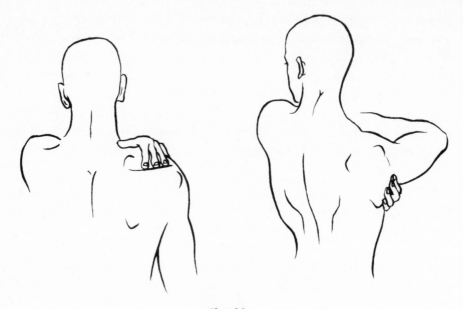

Shoulder

Bottom corner of the shoulder blade (inferior angle).   Follow the "outer edge of the shoulder blade" down to where it ends. You will feel the bottom corner of the shoulder blade move if you raise and lower your arm.

Vertebrae of the neck and upper back (C1–C7, T1–T12).   The bony bumps of the spine. T refers to the trunk (thorax). The vertebrae are numbered from the top down. T1 is the bony bump below the last and biggest bump of the neck (C7), and T12 is right above your waist.

The Rotator Cuff

The four muscles that surround the ball-and-socket joint of the upper arm bone and the shoulder blade are called the rotator cuff muscles. They all attach around the top of the upper arm bone and lie on each side of the shoulder blade, providing strength and support for this joint. It is beneficial to know these muscles: supraspinatus (lifts the arm out to the side and up), infraspinatus (outwardly rotates the upper arm), teres minor (same), and subscapularis (inwardly rotates the upper arm). These muscles are not included in this book.

Shrugging the Shoulder 1 (Shoulder Elevation)

The trapezius is a large, flat muscle that drapes like a cape over the neck and shoulders. It belongs with the neck, shoulder, and upper back muscles and has three parts that relate to different functions: the upper, middle, and lower trapezius. Trapezius means *a shape that has four sides, only two of them parallel.*

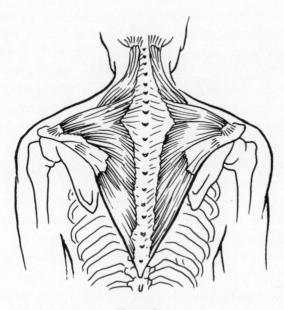

Trapezius

Job

Lifts the shoulders, as in shrugging (upper and middle part; elevation).

Holds the shoulder blade steady while the arm moves (fixation).

Depresses the shoulder (lower part).

Helps to pull the shoulder blade in toward the spine (middle and lower part; adduction).

Also:

Helps to rotate the head and neck far to the opposite side (upper trapezius—one muscle only).

Helps to bend the head, neck, and upper back backward (upper trapezius; extension).

How to Find It

Upper trapezius: To find the beginning tendons, place your fingers in the back center of your skull. Here are two tendons, one on each side of the exact middle of the neck, that feel like soft bumps on the bone. You can feel the pull on the tendons when you bend your neck forward. This part of the trapezius also begins on vertebrae C1 to C5 of the neck. The muscle belly, which often creates a bulge between the neck and the shoulder, spreads out and wraps forward over the edge of the "collarbone" on each side. You can feel it by gliding your hand up and down between the shoulder and the side of the neck.

To find the ending tendon, place your fingers on the last two inches of the "collarbone" before the "tip of the shoulder joint." Press in on top of and in front of the bone and feel the tendon as a squishy band on the bone.

Middle trapezius: To find the beginning tendon, reach one hand over your shoulder and press in along the vertebrae of the upper back (T1–T6). The belly extends out to the side and onto the shoulder.

To find the ending tendon, reach one hand over the opposite shoulder, place it on your shoulder blade, and feel the "upper edge of the shoulder blade" going out toward the shoulder. Press in on and above the bone the last couple of inches before you reach the "tip of the shoulder joint" and feel the tendon as a squishy band on the bone (another great spot to massage).

Lower trapezius: To feel the beginning tendon, place your hand at the back of your waist and, if you can reach, move your fingers up along the vertebrae of the middle back (T7–T12). You will be surprised at how far down this neck and shoulder muscle extends—T12 is almost at the waist! The muscle belly angles in a V shape from the shoulders, with the tip of the V on T12.

To find the ending tendon of this part of the muscle, again reach your hand over the opposite shoulder and place it on the "upper inner corner of the shoulder blade." Press in here and move your fingers down about two inches, and you will be on the ending tendon (a great spot to massage).

To Feel the Lower Trapezius Muscle and Tendon Move: Press in on this last tendon attachment while you hold your arm up and out to the side. You should feel the tendon being pulled as you bring your arm around toward the front and across your chest.

To Feel the Upper Trapezius Muscle and Tendon Move.   Place your hands on your neck right along the spine. The muscle extends vertically down the neck from the skull. While pressing in here, rotate your head from side to side.

Typical Traits

Sometimes this muscle becomes so prominent that the shoulders almost resemble a gothic church. Because it lies over your neck, you may feel as if the neck muscles are causing the tension; in fact, this stiffness can instead stem from movement of the arm as the trapezius muscle attempts to hold the shoulder blade stable. The muscle is under considerable stress, as it supports the shoulder blade. If you work requires you to extend your arms in front of your body to lift heavy objects or move them in front of or above you—for example, picking up a heavy wheelbarrow or carrying objects on the shoulder—the trapezius takes a beating. Recent research has shown that the trapezius is also very susceptible to tension from mental activity. Under stress, we usually elevate our shoulders (also this muscle's job).

Improvement Tip: The upper trapezius is a postural muscle, which means it supports your posture in addition to doing its job, and tends to shorten and tighten. Check your shoulder position when feeling stressed. Gentle stretching along with thorough circulation aid can work wonders. The middle and lower parts of the muscle tend to weaken from abuse. Strengthening is very helpful.

Payoff: You can avoid and heal chronic upper back and neck pain and also the headaches that stem from tension in these muscles as well as the shoulders, which are very tender to the touch or any kind of pressure.

Upper Group
Opposing Muscle: In shrugging, the lower trapezius, which depresses the shoulder.

Assisting Muscles: In shrugging, the rhomboids. In bending the head and neck backward, the splenii. In rotating to the far opposite side, the SCM on the same side.

Middle Group
Opposing Muscle: In pulling the shoulder blade in, the pectoralis major, which pulls the arm forward and in at the shoulder.

Assisting Muscles: In pulling the shoulder blade in at the shoulder, the rhomboids.

Lower Group
Opposing Muscle: In depressing the shoulder, the upper trapezius, which lifts the shoulder.

Assisting Muscle: In depressing the shoulder, the latissimus dorsi.

Shrugging the Shoulder 2 (Shoulder Elevation)

The levator scapulae is a flat muscle that lies perpendicular to the spine. Levator refers to *a muscle that lifts another part of the body*, and scapulae means *shoulder blade*.

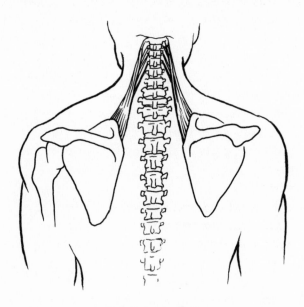

Levator scapulae

Job

Lifts the shoulder (elevation).

Also:

Helps to bend the neck to same side (lateral flexion).
Helps to rotate the head and neck to the same side (cervical rotation).
Helps to bend the neck backward (only slight extension).

How to Find It

Because the tendons begin on the side of the four first vertebrae under the skull, you won't be able to get to them, but you can place your fingers on the side of your neck toward the back, and push in as you move your fingers downward a couple of inches along the sides of vertebrae C1 to C4.

The tendons lie deep inside here. The muscle belly—flat, quite large, and turned sideways—extends down the neck to the shoulder blade.

To find the ending tendon, place one hand over the opposite shoulder. Find the "upper inner corner of the shoulder blade" next to the spine (move your arm to make the corner move). From here, move your fingers up about one and a half inches to feel where this tendon ends. The big shoulder muscle, the trapezius, covers this area, but you can feel through it by pressing a little harder.

To Feel the Muscle and Tendon Move: Place your hand just above the "upper inner corner of the shoulder blade." Position your other hand on the small of your back. Shrug and relax alternately the shoulder whose tendon you are holding while you press in and feel the muscle move as it contracts to lift the shoulder blade. Many people with tense necks and shoulders have bumpy, tender spots in this muscle.

Typical Traits

The levator scapulae, like the trapezius, is located in the neck but primarily moves the shoulder blade. It can get stressed during lifting, especially if your shoulders are hunched or shrugged, because it prevents the shoulder blade from being pulled down when weight is on the arms. It can get even more stressed if you turn your head to one side at the same time. Since it is attached to the joint that rotates the neck (atlas and axis), it is activated each time you turn your head. Following the ball from side to side while watching a game, turning to the side to talk to someone in a seat behind you at the theater, or typing with lifted shoulders while referring to a document located to one side can cause this muscle to give you a stiff neck. It tends to shorten and tighten in reaction to abuse.

Improvement Tip: Check your shoulder position when feeling stressed. Learning to stretch this muscle gently and effectively, along with circulation aid, particularly of the shoulder blade attachment.

Payoff: You can achieve freedom from the most common and painful stiff neck syndrome, which stems from the levator scapulae, and pain while turning the head.

Group

Opposing Muscles: In lifting the shoulder, the lower trapezius and latissimus dorsi, which depress the shoulder.

Assisting Muscles: In lifting the shoulder, the upper trapezius and the rhomboids. In bending the neck to the same side, the scalenes. In bending the neck backward, the splenius cervicis.

Pulling the Shoulders Back (Scapular Adduction)

The rhomboids consist of a minor muscle (upper) and a major muscle (lower), and are located between the shoulder blades and the spine. The name means *shaped like a rhombus.*

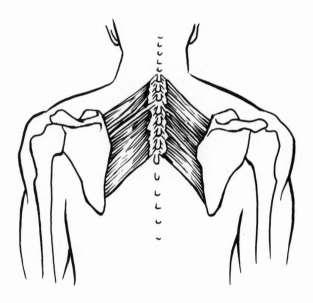

Rhomboids

Job

Pulls the inner edges of the shoulder blades toward the spine (adduction).

Also:

Helps to rotate the shoulder blade so that the lower corner of the shoulder blade moves down and in (downward rotation of the scapula).

Helps to lift the shoulder blades, as in shrugging (elevation).

Helps to fixate the scapula while the biceps and triceps work to lift and straighten the arm.

How to Find It

To find the beginning tendon, place your hand over the opposite shoulder and follow your spine from the top of the neck down to the largest bony bump (C7). Beyond this, on each of the vertebrae down the upper back as far as you can reach (T1–T5), are the beginning tendons. The muscle belly stretches diagonally downward onto the "inner edge of the shoulder blade."

To find the ending tendon, reach your hand over your shoulder blade. Press in with your fingers along the "inner edge of the shoulder blade," and you will feel the tendon.

To Feel the Muscle and Tendon Move: Reach over your shoulder and press in between the shoulder blades, making a strong three-finger push pad. At the same time, bring your other arm, lifted and with elbow bent, across the chest and back several times so that you feel the muscle contract and stretch (small movements are best for feeling the muscle). If you push hard enough, you can feel the muscle belly through the flat trapezius muscle, which covers it.

Typical Traits:

If you reach over and massage between the shoulder blade edges (the tendon site for the rhomboids), you can feel how tender and sore this area often is. It is often necessary to hold your upper arm in front of your body when working for extended periods of time, which puts great stress on the rhomboids, whose job it is to maintain the position of the shoulder blades and draw them together and closer to the spine. These muscles also have to fight the strength of the muscles in front of the shoulder (the pectoralis muscles). They tend to weaken in response to abuse.

Improvement Tip: Straighten your upper body and move your shoulders back. Strengthening.

Payoff: You can straighten your upper back more easily, and start the healing of these often very strained and painful muscles, as well as become free of pain along the inner edge attachment on the shoulder blades.

Group

Opposing Muscle: In pulling the shoulder blades toward the spine, the pectoralis major, which causes the blades to be pulled apart when the shoulders are pulled forward.

Assisting Muscles: In pulling the shoulder blades toward the spine, the middle part of the trapezius. In lifting the shoulder blades, the levator scapulae.

Bringing the Shoulder Blades away from the Spine (Scapular Abduction)

The serratus anterior is like a muscle sheet that wraps around half of the chest in front and under the arm, lying between the shoulder blade and the ribs. It extends under the shoulder blade and attaches to its inner edge, pulling this side of the shoulder blade closer to the ribs. This is how the serratus anterior prevents the shoulder blades from sticking out. The name refers to its shape and location: serratus means *having a sawlike edge* and anterior means *front.*

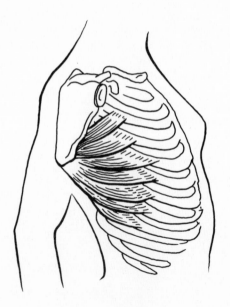

Serratus anterior

Job

Brings the shoulder blades out away from the spine (as in the upward movement of a push-up; scapular abduction).

Also:

Raises the arm high up (more than 90 degrees) in front of the body (scapular abduction).

Pulls the inner edge of the shoulder blades closer to the rib cage, preventing winging (when the shoulder blades stick out and look like wings on your back).

How to Find It

To find the beginning tendon, reach one hand around the opposite side under the arm and place it on the "bottom corner" of the shoulder blade. (You can feel this corner move if you bend your elbow and move it up and down in front of you.) From here, move your hand forward under the arm, halfway toward the center in the front. The muscle's beginning attachments are on the ribs from here up to the collarbone (ribs 1–8; ribs are counted from the top down). The muscle belly lies flat over the ribs along the chest and under the arm. It narrows after rounding the side to end on the inside edge of the shoulder blade. You cannot get to this ending tendon with your hands.

To Feel the Muscle and Tendon Move: Press on the ribs under the arm, from the eighth rib and up, while you move the arm forward and up in front. You should feel the muscle contract.

Typical Traits

You use this muscle when you swim, climb, throw, or shoot in basketball. When you raise the arm forward and up, it moves the shoulder blade forward and up on the rib cage, assisting the arm movement. You rely on it during push-ups. It gets stressed when you hold your arms outstretched in front of your body for extended periods of time as it attempts to keep the shoulder blades fixed on the thorax. In reaction to abuse, it tends to weaken.

Improvement Tip: Correct your posture so the shoulder blades lie flat on your back. Strengthening.

Payoff: You can free yourself of pain in the side under your arm and back under the shoulder blade, and it will be easier to raise your arm forward and up. Also, you will be cured of the winged shoulder blades caused by weak serratus anterior muscles. Stretching can help you get rid of the stitch in the side caused by this muscle that we often experience while running, exercising, or just breathing heavily. Stretching can also help overcome the habit of shallow breathing caused by having a tight serratus anterior.

Group

Opposing Muscles: In moving the shoulder blades forward on the rib cage, the rhomboids, which pull the shoulder blades together. In lifting the arm high up in front of the body, the latissimus dorsi, which pulls the arm backward behind the body.

Assisting Muscles: In lifting the arm high up in front, the pectoralis major. In lifting the shoulder, the upper part of the trapezius.

Raising the Arms (Abduction, Flexion, and Extension)

The deltoid is the muscle that we normally think of as the shoulder muscle, because it wraps around the outside of the shoulder. It is actually three muscles covering the front, middle, and back of the shoulder. Deltoid means *shaped like a delta—a triangle.*

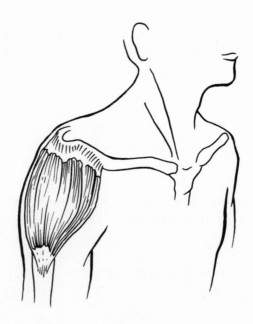

Deltoid

Job

     Raises the arm and shoulder out to the side (middle deltoid; shoulder abduction).

Raises the arm up in front of the body (front deltoid; shoulder flexion and internal rotation).

Raises the arm up behind the body (back deltoid; shoulder extension and external rotation).

How to Find It

To find the beginning tendons for the front, middle, and back deltoids, place your hand on top of the opposite shoulder and press in along and under the last inch of the collarbone, the "tip of the shoulder joint," and the first inch of the "upper edge of the shoulder blade," where the front, middle, and back sections of the muscle begin. While pressing in, move your arm from down at your side in turn to up in front, up in back, and up out to the side. You should be able to feel the tendon stretch during each movement. The muscle bellies cover the whole shoulder and upper arm.

To find the common ending tendon for all parts of the deltoid, place your fingers on the outside of your upper arm, a little less than halfway down the upper arm bone from the shoulder, and press in on the tendon. You can also find this spot if you raise your arm to the side and feel where the muscle bulge narrows on the upper arm. Here is the common tendon.

To Feel the Muscle and Tendon Move: Position your other hand so that it covers your upper arm and feel the muscle contract while you move the arm forward, out to the side, and back.

Typical Traits

The deltoid is one of the most likely muscles to develop pain, but it is also easy to help because you can get at the tendon sites easily, and stretch and strengthen the muscle simply by raising your arm. Lifting the arm out to the side is a typical deltoid action. The muscle is used in any lifting or movement of the arm forward or back, and it always works closely with the rotator cuff muscles. It cannot do any of its jobs without these muscles. The deltoids are strong muscles, but tend to weaken in response to abuse.

Improvement Tip: Strengthening and circulation aid.

Payoff: You can rid yourself of the tension and pain that often build up on the common tendon for all three parts of the deltoid halfway down on the outside of the upper arm. You may find that it no longer hurts to move your arm back and forth, and it will feel comfortable, instead of exhausting, to lift and hold your arm out to the side.

Group

Opposing Muscle: In raising the arm up in front and up behind the body, the deltoid's front and back parts oppose each other. In raising the arm up to the side, the pectoralis major and the latissimus dorsi, which pulls the arm in to the side.

Assisting Muscles: In raising the arm up behind the body, the triceps and the latissimus dorsi.

Rolled-In Shoulders (Flexion, Adduction, and Internal Rotation)

The pectoralis major is a large, thick, fan-shaped muscle that covers the chest, the front of the upper body, and the front of the shoulders. It has an upper and lower part. Pectoralis means *chest or breast*.

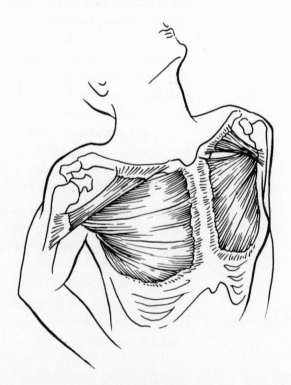

Pectoralis major

Job

Rotates the arm inward (rounded shoulders; adduction, internal rotation).

Pulls the arms to the side and across the chest in front of the body (adduction).

Also:

Helps to raise the arms up in front of the body (upper part of the pectoralis; flexion).

How to Find It

Lower part: To find the beginning tendon, place both hands on your chest at the center on top of the breastbone. Follow the breastbone down, pressing with your fingers on both sides. Press in on each rib, from the top all the way down to the to the sixth rib, right before the breastbone ends. At the same time, extend your arm on the same side in front of you and out to the side as you palpate the ribs, and you should be able to feel the pull on the tendons. The muscle belly covers the chest and narrows at the arm.

To find the ending tendon, place your fingers on the upper arm, in front of your shoulder about two inches down from the "ball on top of the upper arm." Press in as you move this arm, extended in front of you, out to the side and feel the tendon pulling. This ending tendon is the common ending tendon for both the upper and lower parts of the muscle.

Upper part: To find the beginning tendon, place your fingers on the underside of the collarbones where they meet in front and press along the bone two inches toward the shoulder. The short muscle belly stretches from here across to the shoulder. The ending tendon is the shared muscle anchor described above.

To Feel the Muscle and Tendon Move: Press in on one side of your chest about two inches down from the collarbone and two inches away from the breastbone while you move your arm from an extended position straight in front of you to the side, and from there further toward the back. You can feel the pull on both parts of the muscle right here.

Typical Traits

Many of us have overly strong pectoralis muscles that cause us to have rounded, hunched shoulders and a tight chest, making it very hard to hold the upper body straight. You use this muscle a lot when you work with your arms in front of your body or extended in overhead activities. Typical activities include throwing a baseball (the arm is bent and internally rotated, and the shoulder blade is drawn forward), doing pull-ups and push-ups, or throwing and serving in tennis. Overhead work can be especially stressful. The upper part of the muscle tends to become tight and short in response to abuse. The lower parts tend to weaken in response to abuse and can therefore benefit from strengthening.

Improvement Tip: Straighten your upper back and move your shoulders back. Because this muscle gets a lot of strengthening during daily activities but very little stretching, it helps to do a lot of stretching of the upper part of the muscle and some strengthening of the lower part.

Payoff: You may find that you are able to adopt a posture with a comfortably upright upper back and neck. This will relieve neck and upper back pain. You may find that it is no longer difficult for you to lift a heavy object at or near waist level, or to touch your opposite shoulder with your hand. Commonly experienced feelings of chest pain due to tight pectoralis muscles can be relieved, along with chronic pain in the area around the shoulders.

Group
Opposing Muscle: In rounding the shoulders, the rhomboids, which pull the shoulder blades together.

Assisting Muscles: In lifting the arm up in front, the front part of the deltoid.

Working with the Arms Overhead and Behind the Back
The latissimus dorsi is the largest muscle of the back. It forms a big sheet that covers the lower back from under the shoulder blades down to the hips, yet it is actually a shoulder muscle. Shaped like a fan, it attaches along the spine as well as to the outer ends of several ribs, and it is hard to do anything without activating this muscle. Latissimus dorsi means *widest muscle of the back.*

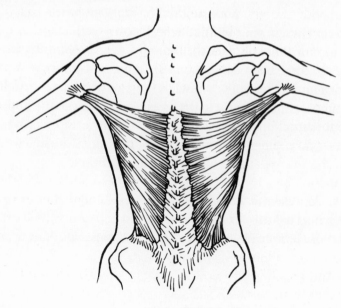

Latissimus dorsi

Job

Pulls the arm back at the shoulder, lifting it behind the body (shoulder extension).

Also:

Helps to roll the arm inward, as used in the crawl stroke while swimming (internal rotation).

Helps to pull the shoulder down and in (shoulder depression and adduction).

Straightens the back as in lifting (hyperextension).

How to Find It

To find the beginning tendon, first note that this large muscle sheet glues to the back, the ribs, the hipbone, the shoulder blade, and the spine, which are all beginning attachments for the latissimus dorsi. Place your hands on your waist with your fingers pointing backward and thumbs facing the front. With your fingers, press along the "hipbone in the back" (ilium), along the vertebrae from the middle back down to the tailbone (T6–T12 and L1–L5), and along ribs 9 to 12, and you will be pushing on the tendon. Along the vertebrae from the hipbone up to the mid-upper back, there are more beginning tendons. The muscle belly covers the lower, middle, and mid-upper back, and from there stretches over, ending at the upper arm.

To find the ending tendon, reach under your armpit and grab your upper arm. The ending attachment for the latissimus dorsi is where your fingers are, on the upper arm bone close to the armpit.

To Feel the Muscle and Tendon Move: Reach under your armpit again and extend your hand as far as you can toward and under the "bottom corner" of the shoulder blade. While facing a wall, raise your free arm up and lean against it, simultaneously pushing on it.

Typical Traits

This muscle covers the entire lower back but is a shoulder muscle. You use it during activities such as climbing a rope, chinning, rowing, or chopping. It acts to lift the body toward the fixed arm just as much as it moves the arm toward the body. In overhead activities, it is stretched under tension. You also use it anytime you move your arm behind your body or whenever the arm is pulled in toward the body or down (depressed). It is naturally a strong muscle, but weakens when it is abused. When it is tight you may have problems lifting your arm forward or out to the side and up. You may be able to notice tightness in the latissimus dorsi by lying on the floor on your back and raising your arm above your head; check to see if your arm will not lie flat on the floor, but instead pulls the elbows out to the side. People who have walked with crutches for a long time often develop shortness in this muscle.

Improvement Tip: Strengthening and stretching.

Group

Opposing Muscle: In depressing the shoulder, the upper trapezius, which lifts the shoulder. In lifting the arm up behind the body, the upper part of the pectoralis major.

Assisting Muscles: In pulling the arm backward, the back of the deltoid and the triceps. In rolling the arm inward, the pectoralis major. In depressing the shoulder, the lower trapezius. In straightening the back, the erector spinae.

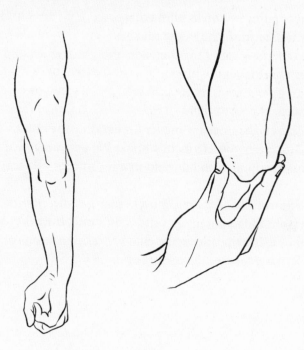

Elbow

Muscles of the Elbow

Bony Landmarks for Locating Muscles that Move the Elbow and the Hand

How to Find Them

Bend your elbow about 90 degrees and bring it across your chest. With your other hand, feel the bony bumps of your elbow; you should feel one large bump with two smaller bumps on each side.

Large middle bump of the elbow (olecranon).   This is the bony bump with which you prop yourself up when you lean your elbow on a table, which actually is the end of the forearm bone on the little finger side (ulna) that extends from your wrist to your elbow and runs parallel with your other forearm bone (radius).

Small outer bump of the elbow (lateral epicondyle).   This is the bony bump located on the outer side of your elbow. It is actually one side of the termination of your upper arm bone, where it ends at the elbow.

Small inner bump of the elbow (medial epicondyle).   This is the bump on the inner side of your elbow that touches your body when you fold your arm across your chest. It is the other side of the upper arm bone, where it terminates at the elbow.

Bending the Elbow (Flexion)

Note: The biceps is the primary mover for bending the arm at the elbow. It is, however, not a key muscle in this book. We encourage you to look up the biceps in other books, find its tendon attachments, and learn about the muscle.

The brachioradialis is a long muscle that lies directly under the skin and reaches from the upper arm to the wrist bone. It works together with the biceps in bending the arm at the elbow. Brachior means *arm* and radialis means *the inner forearm bone on the thumb side.*

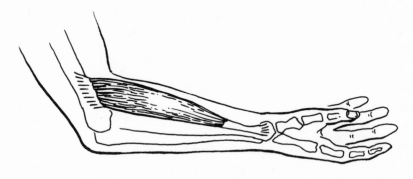

Brachioradialis

Job

Bends the arm at the elbow (elbow flexion).

Also:

Brings the forearm to a position halfway between palms up and palms down.

How to Find It

To find the beginning tendon, place your hand, palm down, on a table in front of you with your arm and elbow outstretched. Place the fingers of your other hand on the outside of your upper arm two inches above your elbow in front of where the triceps tendon passes. You can clearly see the muscle belly as a bulge that passes over the elbow joint and then extends down the forearm to the wrist.

To find the ending tendon, place your fingers on your wrist, just below the bony bump on the thumb side. The tendon attaches deep in this bony area.

To Feel the Muscle and Tendon Move: While your arm is hanging down relaxed at your side, place your fingers on the bulge near the elbow, a little below the beginning tendon. Press in deeply and feel the muscle move as you bend and straighten your elbow. You can also grab the bulge between your fingers and feel the belly tighten as you rotate the arm.

Typical Traits

Many keyboard workers experience pain in this muscle as well as pain from the wrist-lifting (extensor) muscles. The muscle is continuously contracted when it bends the arm at the elbow. It tends to lose endurance capacity, becoming tight and short from abuse.

Improvement Tip: Straighten your arm often and rotate the forearm to massage and stretch.

Payoff: If you keep it healthy, you can treat and avoid pain that starts at the elbow and spreads to the thumb side of the wrist. You can also avoid false tennis elbow syndrome, a condition in which people experiencing pain in this muscle mistakenly think they have tennis elbow.

Group

Opposing Muscle: In bending the arm at the elbow, the triceps, which straightens the arm at the elbow.

Assisting Muscle: In bending the arm at the elbow, the biceps.

Straightening the Elbow (Extension)

The triceps is a long muscle in the back of the upper arm consisting of three parts or heads: the long, middle, and side parts. Tri means *three* and ceps refers to *heads.*

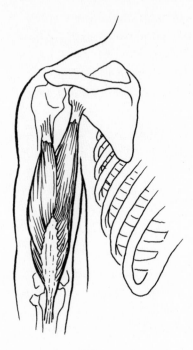

Triceps

Job

Straightens the arm at the elbow (long and side parts; elbow extension).

Also:

Helps to raise the arm up behind the body (long part; shoulder extension).
Stabilizes the elbow while the forearm is turned over, palms down.

How to Find It

Long head: To find the beginning tendon, stretch your arm up above your
head and reach with the other arm under your armpit, placing your fingers
on the "outer edge of the shoulder blade" right at armpit level. Press in
deeply while you bend and straighten the elbow of the raised arm (only
small movements are necessary). You may have to press in around this area
a little to hit the moving tendon. This spot is often sore. The muscle belly
covers the back of the upper arm, all the way down to the elbow.

To find the ending tendon, place your fingers on the "large middle
bump of your elbow" and move up the back of the upper arm about three

inches. You will find a big common tendon where all three parts of the triceps muscle end. The tendon attaches on the "large middle bump of the elbow," but it also goes almost halfway up the back of the arm. You can feel it tighten when you bend and straighten your elbow.

Side head: To find the beginning tendon, place your hand around your upper arm, right below the shoulder, with your thumb toward the front and your fingers around the back of your upper arm. The tendon is deep below your little finger. You can feel it move while you bend and straighten your elbow with your arm raised.

Middle head: To find the beginning tendon, place your hand in the same position as above, but even further down the upper arm—about five inches from the top of your shoulder. Press in deep, to the bone. (This tendon is harder to find.)

To Feel the Muscle and Tendon Move: With a raised arm, press your other hand on the back of your upper arm while you bend and straighten the elbow; you can feel the triceps muscle contract and stretch.

Nerve: The middle and side parts of the triceps lie very close to the radial nerve, which supplies the triceps and the muscles of the hand and fingers. The nerve is vulnerable right at the midpoint of the upper arm bone. If you press hard and long on it there, in severe cases, it can cause you to lose power in the wrist. Also, on the "large middle bump of the elbow" there is a groove where the nerve going to the fingers, the ulnar nerve, runs. Pressing here can give you an electric feeling up and down your arm.

Typical Traits

Are the backs or outsides of your upper arms sore? To understand such upper arm pain, you can check out the extra stress the triceps is under in certain positions due to its two-joint function (the long head crosses the shoulder joint as well as the elbow joint). When your arm is extended forward, the tendon at the shoulder blade is stressed, and when your arm is bent, there is stress on the common tendon at the elbow. Stressed and weak triceps are very common among people who do any kind of work that requires balancing the hands in front of the body with elbows bent, such as keyboard work, sewing, assembly-line work, and playing musical instruments. Unless the triceps is deliberately strengthened, it tends to weaken in response to abuse. It seldom gets the relief of a full stretch during normal activities, nor much strength building. You develop strength in your triceps when you do push-ups thanks to the powerful effects of straightening the arm against gravity, and also, for example, during swimming, boxing, or massage work.

Improvement Tip: Straighten your arm often. Strengthening, circulation aid at the tendon sites, and stretching to relieve tension.

Payoff: By keeping your triceps healthy, you are helping the flow of blood and nerve stimulus to the rest of the arm, including the hand and wrist, thereby preventing problems here as well as relieving the pain in the upper arm. Another sore spot you can relieve is the site where the common tendon for all three anchors to the back of the elbow. You may also find that problems you have had using your upper arm—for example, reaching up to a high shelf with a heavy object in your hand—will be gone, because the triceps regained its health.

Group

Opposing Muscle: In straightening the arm at the elbow, the biceps (not a key muscle) and the brachioradialis, which bends the arm at the elbow.

Assisting Muscles: In lifting the arm up behind the body, the latissimus dorsi. In bringing the arm in toward the body, the pectoralis major.

Turning the Forearm Palms Down (Pronation)

The pronator teres is a forearm muscle because it moves this part of the arm, yet it also has the effect of turning the hand so that the palm faces down. Pronator refers to prone, which means *turned or rotated face down.*

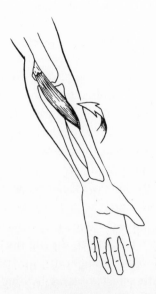

Pronator teres

Job

Rotates the forearm inward, turning the hand palm down (pronation).

Also:

Helps to bend the arm at the elbow (flexion).

How to Find It

To find the beginning tendon, place your forearm on a table with the palm facing up. Place the thumb of your other hand near the elbow, just below the "small inner bump of the elbow" and about an inch toward the inside of the elbow. Here is a big common tendon for the pronator teres and all the muscles that bend the hand and fingers. You can feel it move when you rotate your forearm inward to a palm-down position. The belly extends down the forearm under other muscles as it crosses toward the thumb-side forearm bone. The ending tendon is covered by other muscles in the middle of the "forearm bone on the thumb side," so you cannot feel its attachment.

To Feel the Muscle and Tendon Move: Press in with your thumb just below where you found the beginning tendon while you rotate your forearm so that the palm faces down. This muscle is hard to isolate because when you perform this action, you also feel the finger-bending muscles move below the pronator teres. Try holding near the beginning tendon again, but this time just bend your fingers toward you, rather than rotating the arm. Feel how these finger-bending muscles move in a slightly different place than the pronator teres.

Nerve: The median nerve passes right through the two parts of this muscle.

Typical Traits

When you bend your arm at the elbow and touch the back of your hand to your face, you are using both functions of this muscle (bending the elbow and turning the forearm inward). Any time you turn your forearm in and at the same time bend your arm at the elbow, which is an almost universal motion for any occupation, you stress this muscle. If your arm is turned forcefully, it is powerfully stressed. But less forceful motions, such as keyboard work, can also put considerable stress on it. This muscle is one of the principal muscles involved in repetitive strain injuries of the hand and forearm. Being a flexor muscle, it tends to become tight and short when strained.

Improvement Tip: Rotate your forearm outward often. Stretching and circulation aid.

Payoff: You can relieve yourself of annoying pain on the inside of your elbow and when turning the forearm palm-up, especially if the hand is in a fist. You can also prevent and heal quite painful forearm conditions, such as pronator teres syndrome, which is pain centered on the inside of the forearm close to the elbow, as well as weakness in the wrist and numbness in the thumb and index finger due to compression of the median nerve.

Group

Opposing Muscles: In rotating the forearm inward and turning the palm down, the supinator, which rotates the arm outward and turns the palm up; the biceps; and the brachioradialis, which brings the forearm to the neutral position.

Assisting Muscle: In rotating the forearm inward, the pronator quadratus (not a key muscle).

Turning the Forearm Palms Up (Supination)

The supinator is a short, flat muscle at the elbow that turns the forearm. Supinator refers to supine, which means *lying on the back, face upward.*

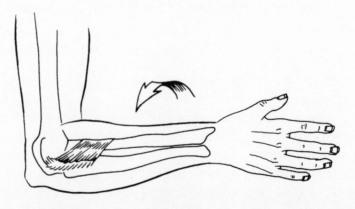

Supinator

Job

Rotates the forearm outward, turning the hand palm up (supination).

Also:

Helps to bend the arm at the elbow when the forearm is in a neutral position (flexion).

How to Find It

To find the beginning tendon, position your forearm palm-down on a table in front of you. Place the fingers of your other hand right below the "small outer bump of the elbow" and press in deeply. You will be pressing on the tendon, which is a common tendon for all the wrist and finger extensor muscles. The short belly of the supinator reaches across the forearm to the "forearm bone on the thumb side." You cannot manually get to the ending tendon because it is covered by other muscles.

To Feel the Muscle and Tendon Move: Hold your fingers on the beginning tendon, as described above, and press in deeply while you rotate your forearm slowly to palm-up. You will feel the overlaying hand and finger-lifting muscles move at the same time as the supinator, which is located underneath them. Next time, try lifting only your hand and wrist instead, without rotating the forearm, and feel the difference in tendon and muscle movement; this time, the supinator is inactive.

Typical Traits

To see this muscle in action, extend your arms straight down in front of you, grasp your hands, and push your straight elbows (elbows only, not your whole arm) forward against the resistance of your grasping hands, turning the forearms outward. Any activity that turns the elbow in this way will contract this muscle. You use it extensively when you turn a screwdriver, carry a briefcase or a diaper bag with your arm straight, or play tennis. It tends to weaken in reaction to abuse and can develop considerable tension.

Improvement Tip: With a straight arm, rotate your forearm inward. Circulation aid and strengthening.

Payoff: You can heal and prevent pain in the elbow due to tiny micro-tears and inflammation of this common tendon (tennis elbow). The supinator is a muscle often involved in tennis elbow syndrome. You also help heal and prevent pronator teres syndrome because you are healing half the problem—namely, the opposing muscle.

Group

Opposing Muscle: In rotating the arm outward and turning the hand palm up, the pronator teres, which rotates the forearm inward and palm down.

Assisting Muscle: In rotating the forearm outward, the brachioradialis.

Muscles of the Hand

Bony Landmarks for Locating Muscles that Move the Wrist

How to Find Them

Outer wrist bump (styloid process of the ulna).   Place your forearm palm-down on a table. Tracing with your fingers, follow your forearm bone—the one on the little finger side closest to the outside of your arm—until you arrive at the point just before your wrist bends. There you can feel a bony bump, the "outer wrist bump," followed by an indentation.

Inner wrist bump (styloid process of the radius).   Keeping your arm in the same position, forearm palm-down on a table, find the bony bump on the thumb side of your wrist, just as you did for the outer wrist bump.

Because the hand muscles have confusingly similar names, keep the following points in mind as you read the next sections: The lifting (extensor) muscles are located on the back of the forearm, one on the little finger side (ulnaris), several in the middle, and one on the thumb side (radialis). These all lift the hand at the wrist (carpi) and fingers (digitorum; from *digiti,* which means fingers). The bending (flexor) muscles are located on the underside of the forearm and correspond in pairs to the lifting muscles on the outside of the forearm, except that there is also a deeper layer of bending muscles. The bending and lifting muscles work together to bend the wrist to the sides.

Bending the Hand (Flexion)

The flexor carpi radialis is a long muscle on the palm side of the forearm. Flexor means *bender,* carpi means *wrist,* and radialis means *on the forearm bone on the thumb side.*

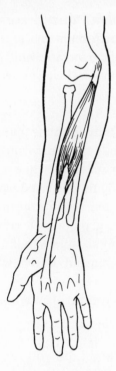

Flexor carpi radialis

Job

Bends the hand at the wrist (flexion).

Also:

Helps bend the hand toward the center, as in reaching for keys in the middle of a keyboard (radial deviation).

How to Find It

To find the common beginning tendon for the finger-bending (flexor) muscles, hold your hand on the table in front of you with the palm facing upward. Place the thumb of your other hand near the elbow, just below the "small inner bone of the elbow" and about an inch toward the middle. Press in here and bend your wrist toward you, and you will feel the tendon. (This is the same common beginning tendon you found for the pronator teres muscle.) The muscle belly extends about halfway down and across the forearm, and becomes a long tendon going to the hand. To find the ending tendons, press in on the base of the index and the middle fingers. This is where the ending tendons attach.

To Feel the Muscle and Tendon Move: Place your fingers on the inside of the forearm, below where you found the beginning tendon. Press in deeply here along the upper third of the forearm while you slowly bend the hand at the wrist. (Slow and small motions help you sense the movement better.)

Typical Traits

This wrist-bending (flexor) muscle on the thumb side has a twin on the little finger side that also bends the wrist. You use these muscles anytime your wrist is bent, curled, or stabilized while you work, normally continuously throughout the day. Thus, the hand- and finger-bending muscles have the endurance capacity required for the many kinds of gripping activities we perform: bicycle riding, motorcycle riding, operating a drill, or any gripping activity such as using scissors, handling heavy tools, or gardening. Still, these fibers tend to tighten and shorten when overly strained.

Improvement Tip: Extend your wrist and rotate the hand often. Stretching and circulation aid.

Payoff: There are many conditions you can heal or prevent that stem from tension in this muscle. Because it attaches to the "small inner bump of the elbow," this common—and commonly painful—tendon contributes to pain on the inside of the elbow and forearm, such as golfer's elbow. You can relieve this, which can cause weakness in the fourth and fifth fingers, burning pain, and a feeling of numbness, as well as pain when rotating the forearm palms up while the hand is lifted backward (extended).

Taking care of the twin muscle, the flexor carpi ulnaris, can help you avoid pains from a condition called Guyon's syndrome, which is due to compression of the ulnar nerve within a canal in the wrist (Guyon's tunnel) that tendons pass through. Also relieved is cubital tunnel syndrome, which causes pain in the elbow by compressing the ulnar nerve between the "small inner bump of the elbow" and the "large middle bump of the elbow."

Group

Opposing Muscles: In bending the hand at the wrist, the extensor carpi radialis (not a key muscle) and the extensor carpi ulnaris. In pulling the hand sideways toward the thumb side, the flexor carpi ulnaris (not a key muscle), which pulls the hand sideways toward the little finger side.

Assisting Muscles: In bending the hand at the wrist, the flexor carpi ulnaris and the flexor digitorum. In pulling the hand sideways toward the thumb side, the extensor carpi radialis.

Lifting the Hand (Extension)

The extensor carpi ulnaris is a long muscle on the back of the forearm. Extensor means *stretch out or lift,* carpi means *wrist,* and ulnaris means *on the side of the ulnar bone* (the forearm bone on the little finger side).

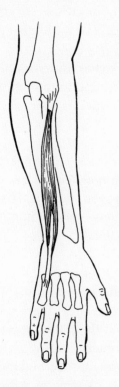

Extensor carpi ulnaris

Job

Lifts the hand at the wrist (extension).

Also:

Helps to pull the hand sideways, as in reaching for distant keys on the sides of the keyboard (ulnar deviation).

How to Find It

To find the common beginning tendon for all the hand-lifting muscles (extensors), place one hand palm-down on a table in front of you and place the other hand on the forearm just below the elbow. As you did when finding the supinator beginning tendon, press in with your fingers just below the "small outer bump of the elbow" and a little toward the middle of the arm (next to the brachioradialis bulge). If you lift your wrist up and down without lifting your forearm, you should feel a tendon moving inside, often tight and ropy. Try to feel the different muscles working (using the same tendon) when you alternate between lifting only the fingers and only the wrist. The muscle belly extends down the forearm toward the wrist.

The ending tendon stretches under a fibrous band at the wrist and attaches on the back of the hand to the first knuckle of the fifth finger. Because of the bones and knuckles, you cannot clearly feel this attachment.

To Feel the Muscle Move: Place your fingers on the upper third of the forearm, just below the beginning tendon, and press your fingers in deeply while at the same time lifting your wrist and hand. You will feel the muscle belly moving under your fingers. Even if it is sore, do not hesitate to push into it; you are stimulating blood flow.

Typical Traits

This is a powerful wrist-lifting (extension) muscle that works together with the smaller muscle on the little finger side, and they both attach on the same common tendon at the elbow. Besides being used anytime you lift the wrist, which is normally continuously throughout the day, you also use it when you perform sudden braking motions with your wrist, such as hitting a tennis ball, digging, or any muscle activity to stop the wrist. This puts a lot of stress on this muscle, which tends to weaken in response to abuse.

Improvement Tip: Bend your hand often and make rotational motions. Circulation aid and strengthening.

Payoff: You will avoid weakness in the wrist and pain on the little finger side of the wrist, and also help prevent or heal tennis elbow syndrome on the common tendon.

Group

Opposing Muscles: In lifting the hand at the wrist, the flexor carpi ulnaris (not a key muscle), which bends the hand at the wrist; the flexor carpi radialis.

Assisting Muscles: In lifting the hand at the wrist, the extensor digitorum. In pulling the hand sideways toward the little finger side, the extensor carpi radialis (not a key muscle).

Tensing the Palm

The palmaris longus is a long muscle of the forearm that has a wide, flat, fibrous tendon that glues to the palm of the hand and narrows into one tendon at the wrist and the forearm. Palmaris refers to the *palm* and longus to the *long muscle going from the palm to the elbow.*

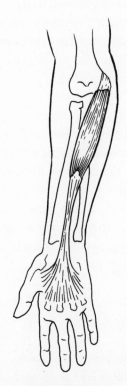

Palmaris longus

Job

Makes the hand into a claw.

Also:

Helps to bend the hand at the wrist (flexion).

How to Find It

Find the common beginning tendon for the hand-bending (flexion) muscles on the "small inner bump of the elbow." You can feel the pull on the tendon if you slowly cup your hand and bend it toward you at the wrist. The belly extends down the forearm close to the little finger side and crosses over toward the middle of the forearm near the wrist.

To find the ending tendon, make a claw with your hand. The tendon, which ends on the base of each finger, narrows into a single tendon at the wrist that you can see on most people and feel if you hold your hand in a claw with your palm facing you. Place your thumb on the inside of the wrist between the "outer and inner wrist bumps," a little closer to the inner. It is the most prominent tendon on the wrist because it does not go under the fibrous band like the finger-bending tendons do.

To Feel the Muscle and Tendon Move: Press in deeply at the common tendon near the elbow while you slowly make a claw with your hand and bend the wrist toward you. This muscle's movement is hard to isolate from the other flexor muscles because it performs the same function, bending the fingers and bending the wrist. (Some people do not have this muscle. Then the other flexor muscles take over this job.)

Typical Traits

This muscle is different from the two other wrist-bending muscles in that it only bends and does not move the wrist to either side. Being a flexor muscle, it tends to become tight and shortened when strained.

Improvement Tip: Spread your fingers often. Stretching and circulation aid, particularly in the palm.

Payoff: By treating this muscle, you can avoid and prevent sore and tender palms that will hurt when you hold tools and contribute to golfer's elbow from tension at the common tendon at the inside of the elbow. You can prevent and also help to halt and heal a condition with a contracture of the tendon of this muscle, which forms the tissue in the hand (Dupuytren's contracture). A little lump in the palm of the hand can develop and attach to the flexor tendon of the fourth finger, which, if allowed to develop, can eventually force the fourth finger into a permanently bent position.

Group

Opposing Muscles: In bending the hand at the wrist, the extensor carpi radialis (not a key muscle), the extensor carpi ulnaris, and the extensor digitorum, which all lift the hand at the wrist.

There is no opposing muscle for the claw-making action.

Assisting Muscles: In bending the hand at the wrist, the flexor carpi radialis and the flexor digitorum.

Bending the Fingers (Flexion)

The flexor digitorum is a long muscle on the inside of the forearm that bends the fingers. Flexor means *bender,* and digitorum refers to the *fingers* or *digits.*

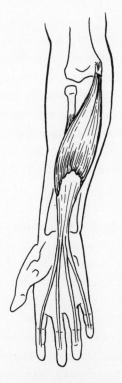

Flexor digitorum

Job

Bends the fingers (flexion).

Also:

Helps to bend the wrist.

How to Find It

Find the common beginning tendon for the finger- and wrist-bending muscles on the "small inner bump of the elbow." The muscle belly extends down the middle of the forearm and splits into several tendons that pass under the fibrous band at the wrist. You can feel the ending tendons on and along the palm side of the fingers and deep in the palm, underneath the palmaris longus muscle.

To Feel the Muscle and Tendon Move: Place your thumb near and just below the beginning tendon, and press while you slowly ball the fingers into a fist. (Slow movements help you sense the muscle better.)

Typical Traits

The finger flexor muscles are the troublemakers in the forearm, the elbow, and the wrist. Every time you bend your fingers you use these muscles, which means most of the time during a person's workday. Any squeezing, gripping, holding, or finger-bending activity uses these muscles. Repetitive kinds of work with little or no full stretching or strengthening especially stress them. They tend to become tight and shortened when strained.

Improvement Tip: Straighten your fingers often. Stretching and circulation aid.

Payoff: If you knew how much trouble you could save yourself by keeping these muscles healthy, you would start right now. By routinely stretching and treating these muscles—paying close attention to the tendon attachment sites, in particular the common tendon—you can prevent and heal pain on the inside of the wrist. Such pain can be caused by compression of the median nerve that goes through the wrist tunnel, the carpal tunnel, which can involve all fingers when allowed to develop, including the thumb. Swelling of the fingers' flexor tendons makes less room for the median nerve as it passes through the tunnel (carpal tunnel syndrome). This pain can be very intense and cause weakness in the wrist. By treating this muscle you can also avoid and treat a variety of other syndromes, such as strain, fiber tear, swelling of the tendon sheaths, and inflammation and strain of the tendons on the "small inner bump of the elbow," which are the symptoms of golfer's elbow. You can also heal and prevent trigger finger, a thickening of the flexor tendon sheath of the middle and ring finger, which often develops nodules inside it that prevent straightening of the finger. The tendon then makes a snapping sound when it passes through the sheath.

Group
Opposing Muscle: In bending the fingers, the extensor digitorum, which lifts the fingers up and backward.

Assisting Muscles: In bending the fingers, the flexor digitorum. In bending the wrist, the flexor carpi ulnaris and the flexor carpi radialis.

Lifting the Fingers (Extension)
The extensor digitorum is a long muscle that lies in the middle of the back of the forearm between the two extensor carpi muscles (ulnar and radialis). Extensor means *stretch out* and digitorum refers to the *fingers* or *digits*.

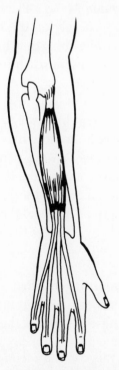

Extensor digitorum

Job

Lifts the fingers up and backward (extension).

Also:

Helps to lift the wrist.
Spreads out the ring, index, and little fingers (abduction).

How to Find It

Find the common beginning tendon for the hand-lifting and finger-lifting muscles on the "small outer bump of the elbow." If you rub back and forth across that spot with the fingers you are pressing in with, you will feel the tight, ropelike tendon. The muscle belly goes down the forearm and splits into several tendons that pass under the fibrous band at the wrist.

To find the ending tendon, place your fingers on the back of the hand and feel the stringy tendons that go to the first row of finger knuckles and continue out the length of the fingers. (These are harder to feel in the fingers, but are on top of the bone.)

To Feel the Muscle and Tendon Move: Place your fingers on the upper third of the forearm. Press in deeply on the forearm an inch and a half below the beginning tendon while lifting only the fingers backward. (Lifting only the fingers helps to isolate this muscle from the wrist-lifting muscle.)

Typical Traits

The extensor muscles are different from the flexor muscles. They are originally strong muscles, but have little endurance capacity. These muscles are not designed for the usage modern work patterns demand, with a huge amount of repeated fine movements of the hands and fingers. Therefore, repeated motions for hours on end without breaks strain, weaken, and tense them. Often the strength of the flexor, overly developed from much usage, causes an imbalance between these two coworkers and the extensor muscles suffer extra strain.

Improvement Tip: Curl your fingers often. Circulation aid of the common tendon where all five major finger-lifting (extensor) muscles attach, gentle stretching until the muscle is healed, then strengthening.

Payoff: By taking care of this common tendon and the muscle, you can heal and prevent pain and weakness in the elbow and weakness of finger grip. You will be able to control the painful inflammation and fiber tearing (tendinitis) that are typical of tennis elbow. Problems with the flexor and extensor muscles of the forearm often go hand in hand. If you have problems with one side, therefore, it is wise to treat the other side also.

Group
Opposing Muscle: In lifting the fingers up and backward, the flextor digitorum, which bends the fingers downward.

Assisting Muscles: In lifting the index finger, the extensor indicis (not a key muscle). In lifting the little finger, the extensor digiti minimi (not a key muscle). In lifting the ring and middle finger, there are no assisting muscles. In lifting the wrist, the extensor carpi ulnaris and the extensor carpi radialis (not a key muscle).

Reaching the Thumb up and out to the Side (Extension and Abduction)

The extensor and abductor pollicis longus are two muscles that move the thumb out to the side and up. Extensor (extend) means *stretch out,* abductor (abduct) means *lead away from the middle,* and pollicis means *thumb* or *big toe.*

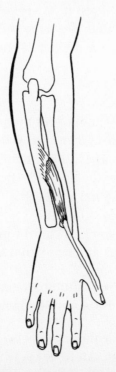

Extensor pollicis longus

Job

Extensor pollicis: Lifts the thumb (palm down) (extension).
Abductor pollicis: Moves the thumb to 90 degrees away from the
 index finger (palm down; abduction).

Also:

Helps to pull the wrist inward, as in reaching to the center (palm
 down; radial deviation).

How to Find It

To find the beginning tendons, hold your forearm palm-down in front of
you, and place your other hand over the forearm below the elbow. With
your fingers, follow the "forearm bone on the little finger side" halfway to
the wrist and move the fingers in about an inch toward the middle. This
thumb tendon attaches here.

The muscle bellies cross over the forearm and end on a tendon on the
base of the back of the thumb (abductor pollicis longus) and along the
thumb (extensor pollicis longus).

To Feel the Muscles Move: Press in where you found the beginning tendon while you lift your thumb up from the table. You should easily be able
to feel the muscle moving. If you don't feel it right away, move your fingers
around the area until you do.

Typical Traits

Try to imagine functioning without your thumb while combing your hair,
shaving, or turning a key in a door and you will understand how much you
depend on pain-free, strong, and healthy thumb muscles. The muscles that
make the thumb reach out to the side and up (palm-up) are used anytime
you hold something that requires a wide grip. They get especially stressed
during work that requires a forceful hand grip, such as grasping large tools,
climbing, or reaching for a complex chord while playing the piano. These
muscles tend to become weak and tense from abuse.

Improvement Tip: Relax your thumb often. Circulation aid of tendon
sites, stretching to relieve tension, and strengthening.

Payoff: Taking care of your thumb extensor muscles can relieve you of
lower forearm pain from the wrist midway up the forearm, including
swelling and pain over the wrist on the thumb side and up the forearm

that increases when you deviate the wrist toward the little finger side (de Quervain's disease).

Group

Opposing Muscle: In lifting and extending the thumb out to the side, the adductor pollicis, which bends the thumb and brings it in across the palm.

Assisting Muscle: These two muscles assist each other in lifting and extending the thumb out.

Moving the Thumb Across the Palm (Adduction)
The adductor pollicis muscle fills the palm between the thumb and the index finger. Adduct means *pull toward the middle,* and pollicis means *thumb or big toe.*

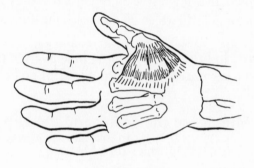

Adductor pollicis

Job
Brings the thumb in across the palm (adduction).

How to Find It
To find the beginning tendon, place your hand palm-up on the table. Using the thumb of your other hand, push on the palm side of the first knuckle of the thumb. The beginning tendon is located here. The muscle belly fills the space between the thumb and the index finger in the palm. You can find the ending tendon between the base of the thumb and the palm along the bone of the third finger.

Typical Traits
The thumb's motion across the palm is as vital as the motion away from it. It is stressed during forceful gripping and hand-twisting while, for example, sewing, hammering, cutting, butchering, playing a musical instru-

ment, sanding or polishing, writing by hand, and weeding. These muscles tend to tighten and tense from abuse.

Improvement Tip: Point your thumb out to the side often so it and the index finger form a right angle. Stretching and circulation aid.

Payoff: You can relieve the ball of your thumb from intense pain and tightness, clumsy hands, problems holding scissors or a pen, clumsiness with any handwork, pain in the palm (weeder's thumb), and trigger thumb, a condition in which you cannot stretch your thumb out without help by the other hand, because the thumb flexor tendon gets trapped as it passes through the adductor muscle in the palm and locks the thumb in flexion.

Group

Opposing Muscles: In bringing the thumb in across the palm, the extensor pollicis and abductor pollicis, which lift and reach the thumb out to the side.

Assisting Muscle: In bringing the thumb in across the palm, the opponens pollicis (not a key muscle) assists the adductor pollicis.

Muscles of the Trunk and the Hip

Bony Landmarks for the Muscles that Move the Back, the Abdomen, and the Hips

Because most of your trunk muscles also attach to your hip, the important bony landmarks for the trunk muscles are found on the hipbone. Form a mental image for a moment of your hipbone, shaped like a bowl. The landmarks consist of the upper rim of the bowl to the side, the front, and the back, as well as the lower rim of the bowl in the front and the back.

How to Find Them

Side of the hipbone (iliac crest). Place your fingers on each side just below your waist and press in. You will feel a bony ridge, which marks the upper rim of the side of the hip bowl.

Front of the hipbone (anterior superior iliac spine). Trace the upper rim of your hipbone around the side toward the front of your body and feel it come to an end about halfway to your navel. Place your fingertips here. If you lean back and a little to one side, you will feel this bone becoming prominent under your fingers.

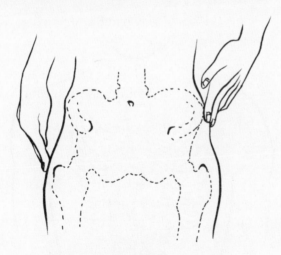

Bony landmarks of the hip region

Back of the hipbone (ilium and sacrum). Follow the "side of the hip-bone" toward the back, where it arches down onto the tailbone at the center of your lower back. Pressing in, you should feel a hard bone about two inches wide, a triangular bone that forms the center back of the hip bowl.

Pubic bone. Position your fingertips at the center of your lower abdomen. The pubic bone is the lowest bony part of the hip bowl.

Vertebrae of the lower back (T12, L1–L5). Feel the bumps of the vertebrae of your lower back. Most of your trunk and hip muscles attach to these vertebrae.

Side and top of the thighbone (greater trochanter of femur). Position your fingers on the outside of your thigh, about a hand's length below the side of the hipbone. Press your fingers in as you raise your foot from the floor and rotate your thigh. You should feel the top of your thighbone moving under your hand.

Bending Forward (Flexion)

The rectus abdominis is a long muscle at the front of the abdomen that runs vertically and is divided by three horizontal fibrous bands. These bands can be seen clearly on bodybuilders, where they look like divisions across the abdomen. Rectus means *straight* and abdominis means *stomach.*

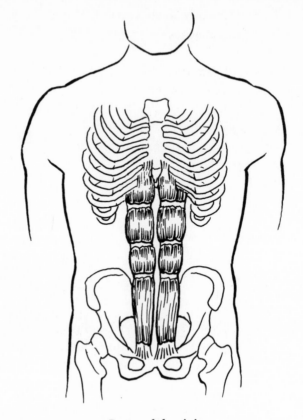

Rectus abdominis

Job

Bends the trunk forward at the waist (sit-up motion; flexion).

Also:

Helps tense the abdominal wall.

How to Find It

To find the beginning tendon, place your fingers at the center of your chest, where the bottom of your breastbone ends and your rib cage splits. There are beginning tendons on the breastbone and on ribs 5 through 7 at the bottom of the breastbone. Press in on the bone and the rib attachments in the triangle here, and you can feel the tendons as slightly squishy bands resting on the bones. If you bend your upper body backward, keeping your hips stable while still pressing in on the bone, you can feel the pull on the tendons. The muscle belly, extending out on each side about one and a half inches from the center, extends down over the stomach to the pubic bone, where the ending tendon attaches.

To Feel the Muscle and Tendons Move: Lie on your back on the floor with your knees bent. Press in on either side of the center of your chest, two or three inches below the triangle where your ribs arch away from the breastbone. Feel the muscle move while you do a slow sit-up motion (you need to make only small movements to feel the muscle contract under your fingers). The other abdominal muscles do not cover the rectus abdominis; so you can get at the tendons and the muscle easily.

Typical Traits

The soft stomach does not feel as if it has much muscle on many of us, yet this long, flat muscle reaching from under the rib cage to the pubic bone is strong when healthy, and also has a significant impact on our bodies. In addition to bending your body forward and getting you out of bed and up from the floor, it helps to hold the abdomen in. When you bend your upper body forward, something most of us do most of the time, the fibers of this muscle are compacted and get very little stretching or strengthening. This muscle tends to weaken from abuse.

Improvement Tip: Adjust your posture to alignment. A slow stretch gives this muscle much-needed circulation aid. Gravity helps to bend the body forward, so the muscle gets little strengthening during the day. Deliberate strengthening is helpful.

Payoff: Not only does your stomach flatten when you strengthen this muscle, but you also relieve tension in your lower back that can accumulate if this muscle is weak. Your abdominal muscles support your postural balance. With normal strength this muscle gives your hip bowl a natural tilt backward (posterior tilt) by pulling tight between the two tendon sites, the breastbone and the pubic bone. When it is weak, however, the pull on the pubic bone is not there, which can cause your hip bowl to tip more forward (anterior tilt) and your stomach to hang out, giving you a sway-back posture. Thus, the benefits of keeping this muscle strong and healthy are many.

Group

Opposing Muscle: In bending the trunk forward, the erector spinae, which straightens the back and bends it backward.

Assisting Muscles: In bending the trunk forward, the iliopsoas. In tensing the abdominal wall, the diaphragm (not a key muscle).

Bending Backward (Extension)

The back muscles are divided into three main groups: muscles whose primary function is to straighten the back, the erector spinae; muscles that primarily rotate it, the transversospinals; and muscles that lie between the vertebrae, the interspinales. The erectors are closer to the surface and the transversospinals are located deeper in the back. We will deal only with the erector spinae here because they are easier to get to, but it is good to keep in mind that under the erector spinae lies a deeper layer of muscles that do much of the work in rotating the back as well as holding it up straight.

The erector spinae: erector means *straight* and spinae refers to the *spine.*

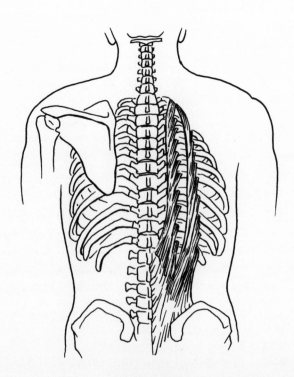

Erector spinae

Job

Bends the trunk backward (extension).

Also:

Helps to bend the trunk to the same side (lateral flexion).
Helps to rotate the trunk.

How to Find It

In the lower back region, the erector spinae muscles are covered by other back muscles, as well as muscles that turn the trunk. However, therapists can work through these intervening muscles to massage the back muscles deeper inside, because they can feel the strong, thick mass of erector spinae muscles underneath. To find the beginning tendon, which is a strong tendon common to all the erector muscles, sit or stand with your hands on the "side of the hipbone," thumbs pointing forward and fingers pointing back and down toward the spine of your lower back. When you extend your fingers so that they are on the "back of the hipbone," which includes your tailbone, you will have found the location of the large tendon that attaches the erector spinae group. (This is a great place to massage!) This muscle also begins on the many vertebra bumps of your lower back (T12 and L1–L5). This is one of the few muscles that begins in several places. The muscle bellies extend from the hips all the way up to the neck, branching out over the ribs in the lower back, the middle back, the upper back, and the neck. As a result, the ending tendons are numerous and attach to all the ribs in a column of tendon attachments that goes up to the neck.

To Feel the Muscle and Tendon Move: Press your finger pads in deeply along both sides of your spine. The muscle is best felt in the mid-lower back, where it is thickest and strongest. Feel the muscle move while you bend your back forward and straighten it up again. You don't have to use big movements to feel the muscle moving.

Typical Traits

These muscles are arranged in one deeper and one more superficial layer that consist of many separate parts woven into a single long muscle sheet that goes all the way from the neck to the hipbone. Because these are postural muscles, stabilizing the back to prevent it from flopping forward, backward, or to the side, as well as moving it, they are in constant use. Anything that happens between the neck and the tailbone affects the entire muscle sheet. Because there is a close interconnection between the many erector spinae muscles, frequently tensing the neck muscles is commonly experienced as pain down in the lower back. When you bend forward, for example, there is a pull on the row of vertebrae as the muscle attaches to the bump of each vertebra. This increases the distance between the bumps when you bend forward and brings them closer together when you straighten your back or bend backward. Sudden trauma and bending and twisting at the same time are common ways to abuse the back muscles, as well as sitting immobile for long hours (for example, on a plane). The lower part of the muscle tends to tighten and shorten in response to abuse, whereas the upper back and neck tend to weaken. Tension is usually felt the most at the huge, strong tendon common to all the back muscles that attaches along the tailbone and the hipbone, causing an aching lower back.

Improvement Tip: Adjust your posture so your body is in alignment. Motion is what gives the back relief, not, as we tend to assume, staying immobile in an attempt to spare it. By intermittently stretching and contracting during the day, giving your back muscles a balanced usage of both, you relieve the fibers. Give the large common tendon a good circulation aid.

Payoff: Learning to treat this tendon can do wonders for your tense back. When, little by little, you stretch and strengthen these muscles, re-teaching the fibers that they can relax as well as contract, you will be rewarded with a reduction of back pain that may surprise you. The long list of symptoms caused by an abused back includes deep, steady aching close to the spine (lumbago), pain in the buttocks, and pain while rising from chairs, going upstairs, or getting out of bed.

Group
Opposing Muscles: In bending the trunk backward, the rectus abdominis and the iliopsoas, which bend the trunk forward.

Assisting Muscles: In bending the trunk backward, the transversospinals group (the deepest layer of back muscles—not key muscles) and the quadratus lumborum.

Bending the Trunk Sideways (Lateral Flexion)
The quadratus lumborum is a muscle that lies deep and close to the spine in the back. It is covered by the erector spinae, but extends out to the sides a little further. Quadratus means *square or rectangular,* and lumborum means *near the loins.*

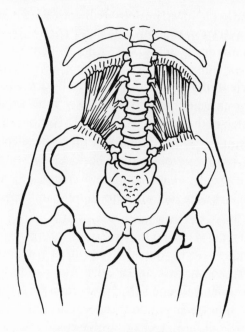

Quadratus lumborum

Job

Bends the trunk to the same side (lateral flexion).

Also:

Helps to bend the trunk backward (extension).
Controls and stabilizes the movement of the same muscle on the
   opposite side of the body.
Tilts the hip bowl to the side.

How to Find It

To find the beginning tendon, place your hands, with thumbs pointing forward and fingers going straight backward, on the "side of the hipbone." The tendons are located on the inner edge of the "side of the hipbone" and extend from where your fingers are in the back and two inches out toward the sides. They are covered by other tendons and muscles, so you cannot get to them. By pushing in deeply and massaging around the site, you can help relieve your lower back of tension. The muscle belly runs parallel with the spine and upward to the ribs.

To find the ending tendon, push in with your fingers on the last rib in the back while bending to the opposite side. The muscle also ends deep along the vertebrae of the lower spine (L1–L4 and T12).

To Feel the Muscle and Tendon Move: Stand sideways on the step of a staircase. Placing your hands on both sides above your "side of the hipbone" and below the last rib in the back, push in deeply. Feel how the muscles move on both sides as you slowly lower one foot off to the step below, lowering your hip, and then raise your foot and hip back up; continue to raise the foot even higher above the step. During this movement, one side works to lift your hip, while the opposite side works to counter and stabilize this motion.

Typical Traits

This muscle strongly affects your ability to hold your body straight and centered, not tilting to one side or the other. You can feel it working deep to the spine as you bend to one side. How often do you bend your body fully to one side? Only when you do this does this muscle get a full stretch. In modern life we don't have large movement patterns, so we usually leave this muscle with very little opportunity to stretch or strengthen during daily activities. Our living patterns, however, do provide conditions for it to become unevenly strong and tight. It tends to shorten and tighten when abused. Habitually leaning to one side while sitting or standing can build tension slowly in the twin muscle, over time making it so tight that it becomes unable to let go. When you suddenly bend widely to one side, the muscle now may not have the strength or health to tolerate the movement and can tighten severely, causing much pain.

Improvement Tip: Make sure you hold your body centered straight and not tilting to the side. Stretching and circulation aid.

Payoff: By treating this muscle, you can gain a feeling of flexibility in your upper body movement, freedom from deep aching along the hipbone in the side and lower back, and also freedom from pain in and right under the lower ribs. You may also discover that what you thought was a leg-length difference (frequently one leg appears shorter than the other if this muscle pulls tighter on one side) is simply tightness in this hip-lifting muscle.

Group

Opposing Muscle: In bending the trunk, the quadratus lumborum on the other side, which bends the trunk to the opposite side and stabilizes the side not bending.

Assisting Muscles: In bending the trunk to the same side, many muscles assist, including the erector spinae and the iliopsoas. In bending backward, the erector spinae.

Muscles of the Hip and the Thigh

The Bony Landmarks for Finding the Hip and Thigh Muscles
How to Find Them
The bony landmarks for locating the hip and thigh muscles are the same as for finding the muscles of the trunk. See page 142.

Bending the Hip (Flexion)
The iliopsoas is the name of two muscles that often are treated as one, consisting of an upper part (psoas) and a lower part (iliacus). The psoas is a long muscle that lies close to the spine in the abdominal area. It joins the tendon of the iliacus, passes in front of the pubic bone, and extends down to the inside of the thighbone. The iliacus is a broad, flat muscle that fills the inside of the hipbone. Psoas refers to *muscle of the loin* and iliacus means *near the ilium* (the top part of the hip bone).

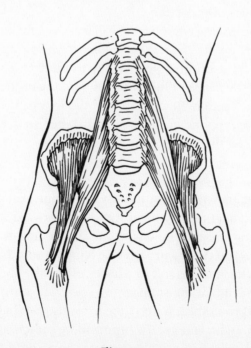

Iliospoas

Job

Bends the body at the hip—the knee toward the chest (hip flexion).
Bends the trunk forward at the waist (trunk flexion).

Also:

Helps to rotate the hip outward (external rotation).
Helps to bend the spine to same side (lateral flexion).

How to Find It

To find the beginning tendon for the upper part (psoas), imagine that you could push in along the spine from directly underneath the last rib and on each vertebra of the abdomen and lower back. This is where the tendons begin. The muscle belly goes down the side of the spine and passes in front of the lower hipbone to the inside of the thigh. It is hard to feel this muscle belly, but being aware of its location is very useful in understanding how to stretch the muscle. This long, narrow muscle ends on the inside of the thighbone. To find the ending tendon, sit on a chair with one leg stretched out forward (foot on the floor) and your upper body leaning back. Place your fingers where the hip bends on the pubic bone and follow this bone to the side, which will take you deep into the groin. Here, both the muscle and the tendon pass over the bone.

To find the beginning tendon for the iliacus, lean forward while sitting. Place your fingers on the "side of the hipbone" and along the ridge going forward to the "front of the hipbone." Try to push in with your thumbs over the ridge to the inside of this bone (as if on the inside of a bowl), and you will be at the tendon attachments for the lower muscle. The muscle extends down the hipbone in the front, joins the psoas, and ends on the common tendon on the inside of the thighbone.

Typical Traits

This muscle is unknown to most of us, yet it is our primary hip-bending muscle. You use it anytime you bend your body forward at the hip. Unlike the trunk-bending stomach muscle, rectus abdominis, it connects to the thighbone. When you raise your leg while lying on your back on the floor, you mostly use this muscle, and to a lesser extent the abdominal muscle. Therefore, to strengthen the stomach muscles, you must lift your trunk instead and bend your knees to relax the hip muscle. When you do sit-ups with your legs straight, you use the hip-bending muscle as well. Sitting all day hurts this muscle, because it is confined in a shortened position for long hours. Ballet dancers often overwork this muscle during repeated leg raising. It tends to tighten and shorten in response to abuse.

Improvement Tip: Stand up and lengthen the front often. Stretching.

Payoff: By taking care of this muscle, you can remove a potent source of lower back pain (forward or uneven tilt of the hip bowl, causing increased or uneven curve) because you are restoring a balanced hip posture. You also rid yourself of the abdominal tightness and groin pain that stem from tightness in this muscle.

Group
Opposing Muscles: In bending the body at the hip, the gluteus maximus and the hamstrings, which both straighten the hip.

Assisting Muscles: In bending the hip, the rectus femoris (one of the quadriceps), the tensor fasciae latae, and the adductors. In bending the trunk to the same side, the quadratus lumborum.

Straightening the Hip (Extension)
The gluteus maximus is the big muscle that covers the buttocks. Gluteus means *rump* or *buttocks* and maximus means *large.*

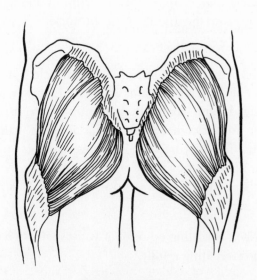

Gluteus maximus

Job
Straightens the body at the hip (extension).

Also:

Helps rotate the thighs outward (external rotation).
Helps to pull the thighs together (adduction).
Stabilizes the knee.

How to Find It
To find the beginning tendon, place your hands on the "side of the hip-bone" with your thumbs pointing forward and your fingers pointing back and down toward the "back of the hipbone." The gluteus maximus attaches on the tailbone and along part of the hipbone. You should feel the pull on the tendon when you press in and slightly under the hipbone in the buttocks (the edge of the hip bowl in the back, going from the tailbone to the "side of the hipbone") while you bend forward at the hip. (Only small movements are needed.) The muscle belly covers the buttocks and narrows onto the thigh. To find the ending tendon, place your fingers on the "side and top of the thighbone" about a hand's length down from the waist. Here and below, the muscle inserts into the long, strong sheath of connective tissue (iliotibial band) that runs down the side of your thigh to the knee. You can feel this tendon on the side of the thighbone.

To Feel the Muscle and Tendon Move: While walking up stairs, press your fingers deeply into the middle of the buttocks.

Typical Traits
This muscle is the principal hip-straightening muscle, but is just as important for the lower back, as it maintains a balanced, upright posture. It holds the hip bowl steady and centered, preventing it from tilting forward. Sitting on your buttocks keeps this muscle in a half-stretched and compressed state. Considering how much we need its strength while we run, hop, return to a standing position from squatting, swim, skip, climb, and jump, keeping it healthy is a good investment. This muscle tends to weaken in response to abuse.

Improvement Tip: Standing up often if you usually sit a lot, strengthening exercises, and stretching it fully.

Payoff: If you take care of this muscle, the pain you may experience while sitting or walking uphill or while swimming may go away and you will be able to go hiking while suffering less soreness in the buttocks afterward. You will receive good support for your lower back, and prevent the lower back strain and pain stemming from this source.

Group

Opposing Muscles: In straightening the hip, the iliopsoas and the rectus femoris (one of the quads), which bend the hip at the thigh.

Assisting Muscles: In straightening the hip, the hamstrings and the erector spinae. In rotating the thigh outward, the piriformis. In moving the thighs together, the adductors.

Rotating the Legs Outward (External Rotation)

The piriformis is a thick, short, flat, and broad muscle located inside the buttocks and has approximately the form of a pear. Piri means *pear* and formis refers to *shape.*

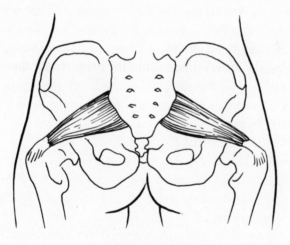

Piriformis

Job

Rotates the thigh out to the side (external rotation).

How to Find It

The beginning tendon is located on the tailbone, inside the hip, so you won't be able to get to it with your hands. The muscle belly is short and broad and reaches out through the hipbone to end on the thighbone. To find this ending tendon, place your fingers on the "side of the hipbone" and move down to the "side and top of the thighbone," about a hand's length down, as you did with the gluteus maximus. Several important muscles attach here, and you may find that this is a sore spot.

To Feel the Muscle and Tendon Move: Push in deeply on the back of the "side and top of the thighbone" bump while you rotate the leg outward. (You will feel the gluteus medius move at the same time because it shares this job.)

Nerve: Passing right under the piriformis muscle, the sciatic nerve supplies the back of the thigh, the leg, and the foot. Also passing through here are the nerves that supply the gluteus maximus, the gluteus medius, and the tensor fasciae latae, as well as the nerve that supplies many of the major pelvic floor muscles. It is very important for the health of the hip, the pelvic floor, the thigh, and the foot that these nerves function normally. If the piriformis is tight, it can put pressure on some or all of these nerves and also on the blood vessels in the area.

Typical Traits

To check if your piriformis muscle may be abused during your daily activities, notice where and how your legs are positioned when you are sitting comfortably at work or while driving your car. Determine if your thighs are apart, knees and/or feet turned out to the side. Every time your thigh is turned (rotated) out to the side, you contract the piriformis, and every time you turn it inward, you stretch it. The muscle is deep inside the buttocks, along with five other hip-rotator muscles. Any kind of pedal work in which the pedal is positioned to one side of the body can cause you to overuse these muscles—for example, when you twist your foot to step on the gas pedal, or when you use a sewing machine for hours without a break. Many other activities do this also, such as ballet dancing, swinging a baseball bat, or taking off on one leg, suddenly externally rotating the hip. These muscles tend to tighten and shorten in response to abuse.

Improvement Tip: Limit rotation of your leg. Stretching and circulation aid at the tendon site on the thighbone.

Payoff: If you have had deep buttock pain combined with hip pain, and/or pain along the entire back of the thigh and the foot, relieving this muscle may get right to the core of your pain problem. The intense pain you may have had directly above the "side and top of the thighbone" may diminish. If you have been unable to fully turn your foot inward, this limitation will end. Pain that occurs when you move the thigh out to the side while sitting, along with lower back pain, may be reduced, as well as pain in the groin, the leg, and the foot. (Ballet dancers who walk with their feet turned out often have such tight and strong external hip rotators that their feet can no longer turn inward or straight ahead. They often experience intense hip pain in the buttocks, which can be relieved through stretching.)

Group

Opposing Muscle: In rotating the thigh outward at the hip, the gluteus medius—the front part rotates the thigh inward.

Assisting Muscles: In rotating the thigh outward at the hip, the gluteus maximus and a group of short rotator muscles located right under the piriformis.

Pulling the Legs Together (Adduction)

The adductor longus, magnus, and brevis muscles are grouped together because they have the same function. The adductor longus is the most superficial (closest to the surface) of the three, while the adductor magnus is the largest and the deepest. Adduction means *pull toward the middle,* longus means *long,* magnus means *large,* and brevis means *short.*

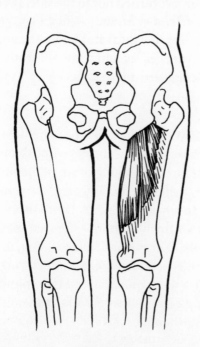

Adductors

Job

Brings the thighs together (adduction).

Also:

Helps to bend the hip (flexion).

How to Find It

To find the beginning tendon, place your fingers on the inside of your thigh, as close to the groin as possible. You should feel a hard string that seems almost like a bone. These are the tendons of the adductor muscles, which begin on the pubic bone in the front. The three muscle bellies extend down on the inside of the thigh and the knee.

The ending tendons are located along the inside of the thighbone. The brevis ends highest on the thighbone; the next one down, the longus, ends about a third of the way down from the pelvis toward the knee; and the magnus ends along the inside of the thighbone on the inside of the knee. Press in just above the inside of the knee and rub your fingers back and forth. Many people have tight tendon attachments here because of tight adductor muscles.

To Feel the Muscle and Tendon Move: While standing, hold and press on the inner thigh of one leg directly at and under the groin while you slowly pull that leg toward the other leg and across in front of it. You should be able to feel the muscle tighten as it contracts.

Typical Traits

Why do the insides of your thighs often become tight and painful? While you sit, the adductors are held in a shortened position with no stretching, and they get very little more stretching or strengthening during daily activities. As you walk, they bring the thighs toward the center, but otherwise do not get much usage. So when you suddenly use them in any activities that include kicking or other thigh motions—for example, swimming (breaststroke and kick), football, horseback riding, skiing, unaccustomed bicycle rides, or when you take a sudden fall or slide, trying to prevent the legs from spreading apart—these muscles are easily injured. Sudden overload and overstretching are common ways to hurt them. They react to abuse with tightening and shortening.

Improvement Tip: Gradual stretching.

Payoff: Your thighs will stop feeling so tight on the inside. Long-term pain you've had in the groin may also go away. Your hip pain will have a chance to heal because the pull on the pubic bone from tight adductors has let go.

Group

Opposing Muscle: In bringing the thighs together, the gluteus medius, which moves the thigh out to the side.

Assisting Muscles: In bringing the thighs together, the gracilis (not a key muscle). In bending the hip, the iliopsoas, the rectus femoris (quads), and the tensor fasciae latae.

Moving the Legs Apart (Abduction)

The gluteus medius is a smaller muscle than the gluteus maximus and covers the side of the buttocks. Gluteus means *rump* or *buttocks* and medius means *middle.*

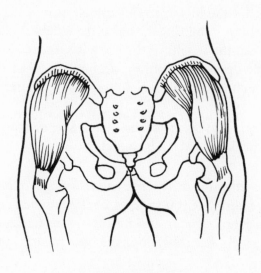

Gluteus medius

Job

Moves the thighs apart (abduction).
Rotates the thigh inward (internal rotation).

Also:

Helps to bend the hip (flexion).

How to Find It

To find the beginning tendon, place your fingers on the "side of the hip-bone." Press in along this edge, which is where the beginning tendon attaches. The muscle belly extends over the side of the hip and reaches down to the thighbone. The gluteus maximus overlays a lot of this muscle except for right at the side. The ending tendon is at the "side and top of the thighbone" and is covered by the gluteus maximus because the two end in the same place.

To Feel the Muscle and Tendon Move: Press into the side on the "side and top of the thighbone" while you move your leg straight out to the side or rotate your hip outward by turning your foot out to the side.

Typical Traits

Every time you put your hands on your hips, you most likely put them on the gluteus medius (and maximus) because it lies directly on the side of the hip, starting on the hipbone. This muscle is in constant use during walking and running, stabilizing the hip as the weight shifts from one side to the other. When the weight of the body is suspended on one leg, the muscle keeps the opposite hip from sagging. You need this muscle for proper alignment. It tends to weaken in response to abuse.

Improvement Tip: Always stretch this muscle after exercise. Strengthening, stretching, and circulation aid if it is painful.

Payoff: By strengthening this muscle and relieving it of pain, you can get rid of pain in the hip while you walk, sit, or sleep on that same side. When treated, the pain at both tendon attachments—sore, tender areas along the "side of the hipbone" (iliac crest) or on the "side and top of the thighbone" may disappear.

Group

Opposing Muscle: In moving the thigh out to the side, the adductors, which bring the thighs together.

Assisting Muscles: In moving the thighs out to the side, the tensor fasciae latae and the piriformis. In rotating the thigh inward, the tensor fasciae latae. In bending the hip, the iliopsoas.

Moving the Hip and the Knee

The tensor fasciae latae is a muscle with a short belly that stops at the top of the thigh and has a tendon that blends with a long tract of connective tissue, the iliotibial band (IT band), that runs down the outside of the leg to the outside of the knee. This band is good to know about because it can become very tense and tight. The tensor fasciae latae muscle is of special interest to us because of its connection with this band and also because it is a two-joint muscle, moving both the hip and the knee. Tensor means *to tense,* fascia means *tissue,* and lateral means *on the side.*

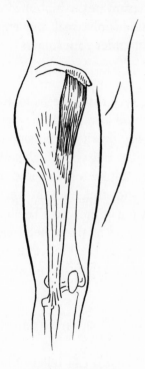

Tensor fasciae latae

Job

Bends the leg at the hip (flexion).

Also:

Helps to move the thigh straight out to the side (abduction).
Helps to rotate the thigh inward (internal rotation).
Helps to bend and stabilize the knee (via the IT band).

How to Find It

To find the beginning tendon, place your fingers on the "front of the hip-bone." The tendon is located on the outside of the front portion of this bone. The short belly extends at a slight angle from the "front of the hipbone" to the outside of the thigh. To find the ending tendon, place your fingers two or three inches below the "side and top of the thighbone." At this point, the tendon mingles with the IT band.

To Feel the Muscle and Tendon Move: While standing, press on the beginning tendon on the "front of the hipbone" while bending your knee or rotating it out to the side (only small movements are necessary). You can feel the muscle moving under your fingers.

Typical Traits

What makes this muscle very different from the gluteus medius, even though it has a similar job and location, is the way it ends in a long, strong tendon that goes all the way down the outside of the thigh to the knee joint. If you have a habit of turning your thigh and foot outward, this muscle works hard to prevent this movement and gets a lot of stress while doing so. When you bend and straighten the knee, the long tendon glides back and forth on the outside of the knee. The long tendon (the IT band) functions as a stabilizing sheet of tissue between the thighbone and the lower leg bone. The muscle is the kind that tightens and shortens in response to abuse. You may find that the entire outside of your thigh feels very tense and painful.

Improvement Tip: Lots of circulation aid and very gentle stretching.

Payoff: Gentle work in this area can relieve hip pain concentrated near the "side and top of the thighbone," as well as outer thigh and knee pain. You can also heal and prevent such painful conditions as runner's knee, which is inflammation of the fluid-filled sac, the bursa, on the outside of the knee due to irritation from the IT band gliding back and forth across the "upper outside bump of the knee," the lateral condyle of the femur. This way, a tight hip muscle, surprisingly, can cause intense pain at the knee.

Group

Opposing Muscle: In bending the hip, the gluteus maximus, which straightens the hip.

Assisting Muscles: In bending the hip, the iliopsoas and the rectus femoris (quads). In rotating the thigh inward, the gluteus medius. In bending the knee, the hamstrings.

Muscles of the Knee

Bony Landmarks for the Muscles that Move the Knee

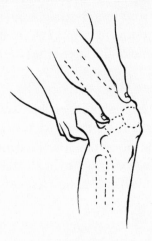

Knee

How to Find Them

The bones are best found sitting with a bent knee. While you sit, feel the kneecap and the bony sides of the knee with your thumbs. The thighbone, the femur, ends at the knee joint, where it is wide and forms two easily recognizable bony landmarks, one upper bump on each side of the knee right above the kneecap. The major muscles of the knee attach to these bumps.

Upper outside bump of the knee (lateral condyle of the femur).
Upper inside bump of the knee (medial condyle of the femur).

Lower down, right under the kneecap, you will find two more bony bumps. These are the two lower bumps at the top end of the shinbone, the tibia. The lowest bump stems from the smaller lower leg bone that runs parallel with the shinbone. Major muscles of the foot and the knee attach to these bumps.

Lower outside bump of the knee (lateral condyle of the tibia).
Lower inside bump of the knee (medial condyle of the tibia).

There is also a smaller lower leg bone, the fibula, located on the outside of the lower leg, which forms yet another bony landmark.

Lowest outside bump of the knee (head of the fibula). Find the lower edge of your kneecap and then continue down about one and a half inches. Move your thumb straight out to the side and you will find a small but prominent bump. It is located right under the "lower outside bump of the knee," the lateral condyle of the tibia.

Bending the Knee (Knee Flexion)

The hamstrings are a group of muscles that work together to bend the knee and extend the hip and are therefore two-joint muscles. The three hamstring muscles are the biceps femoris, the semiteninous, and the semimembranosus. The term *hamstrings* refers to the stringy tendons at the back of the knee that tie the hamlike muscles to the bone, so to speak.

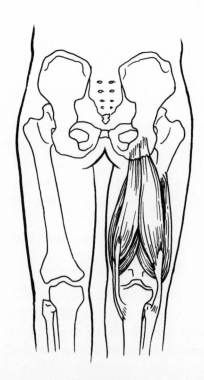

Hamstrings

Job

Bends the knee (knee flexion).

Straightens the hip (hip extension).

How to Find It

To find the beginning tendon, follow the back of the thigh up to the hip bone underneath the buttocks. It is easiest to find this if you bend forward and trace the hard, stringy tendons at the top of the thigh to the buttocks until you find the bone. The tendons attach here, closer to the groin than to the outside, on a common tendon for the three hamstring muscles. (Once you've found it, this is a great spot to put pressure on and massage.) The muscle bellies extend down the back of the thigh and then separate to each side of the knee.

To find the ending tendon of the hamstring on the outside of the thigh—the biceps femoris, which crosses the back of the thigh to the outside of the knee—sit with your knees bent. Feeling underneath the outside of the knee, you will find two very thick, strong tendons. Follow them down the side of the knee and onto the "lowest outside bump of the knee," and also onto the "lower outside bump of the knee," where these tendons attach. Press in just above the bones and you will be right on the tendon attachments for this strong muscle. The two other hamstring muscles run along the inside of the back of the thigh. To find the ending tendons for these, sit with your knee bent and feel underneath the inside of the back of the knee to find another strong tendon. Follow this tendon to the side, where it attaches onto the "lower inside bump of the knee." Press in right above this bone and you will be on the tendon site. Both of the hamstrings on the inside of the thigh attach here. These are great places to massage.

To Feel the Muscle and Tendon Move: While standing, place your hand on the back of your thigh, about one-third of the way down from the buttocks to the knee. Press in here while you bend and lift your knee. (Only small movements are necessary to feel the muscle contract.)

Typical Traits

Many people hate to stretch their hamstrings because it hurts, seems to feel tighter after stretching, and takes too long to get results. This perception is often due to a failure to understand how these hypersensitive, two-jointed muscles work. Gentle stretching is much better than ballistic stretching, which only makes them tighter. Remember that the length and tension monitors respond to the way you stretch. There are many reasons why, for so many of us today, our hamstrings are in bad shape. When sitting, the entire body's weight compresses the underside of your thigh, cutting off blood circulation for hours at a time. The fibers become oxygen-starved, tensed, and often unable to take the load when you need their strength, which is every time you bend your knee. You use these muscles while walking, running, jumping, hopping, climbing stairs, and skipping. Because they move two joints, they are doubly stressed. These muscles tighten and shorten when abused.

Improvement Tip: Stand up and stretch your legs often if you sit a lot. Gentle, careful, and frequent stretching over time until they lengthen; circulation aid, particularly on the many tendon sites in the buttocks and around the back of the knee.

Payoff: By keeping your hamstrings free of tension and shortening, you can avoid multiple and complex pain patterns in the hip and the thigh. Pain in the backs of the thighs while walking and pain in the back of the knee or in the buttocks can be relieved. You will help to relieve lower back and hip pain caused by tight hamstrings that pull the hip bowl too far backward. Also, pain due to unevenly tight hamstrings—pulling more on one side of the hip than the other, leading to many muscle tension conditions—will slowly be relieved. Painful buttocks, hamstring syndrome—a result of tight, possibly inflamed tendon sites where they fit into the hipbone in the buttocks—and pain down the back of the thigh with tender, ropelike bands in the muscle are things you can prevent and relieve. Painful and snapping hamstring tendons on the inside of the knee (one of the hamstrings inserts onto the head of the "lower inside bump of the knee") while bending or straightening the knee can also be cured by treating the muscle and its tendon sites.

Group
Opposing Muscles: In bending the knee, all the quadriceps, which straighten the knee. In straightening the hip, the iliopsoas, which bends the hip.

Assisting Muscles: In bending the knee, the three hamstrings assist each other. In straightening the hip, the gluteus maximus.

Straightening the Knee (Extension)
The quadriceps is a powerful group of muscles on the front of the thigh. They are, in fact, the most powerful muscle group in the human body. We

divide these into two groups: one muscle called the two-joint quad (the rectus femoris) because it works both the hip and the knee joint, and four other muscles called one-joint quads because they work only the knee joint. Quadriceps refers to *a muscle with four heads.*

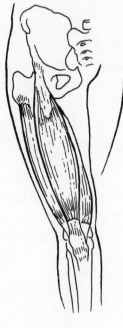

Quadriceps

Job

Straightens the knee (Extension).
Bends the hip (two-joint quad only; hip flexion).

Also:

Helps to ensure the balance of the body by contracting when, for example, bending backward, squatting, and sitting down.

How to Find It

The two-joint quad begins on the hipbone in the front, crosses the hip-thigh junction, and extends down to cross over the patella (kneecap) at the knee joint. To find the beginning tendon, sit on a chair, leaning back with one leg stretched out in front (foot on the floor). Place your fingers on your outstretched leg in the groin area, right where the hip bends at the thigh, about one-third of the way in from the outside of the thigh. Press in deeply while lifting up your leg with a straight knee. You should feel the pull on this strong tendon. The muscle belly stretches down the middle of the front of the thigh. To find the ending tendon, place your thumbs about an inch above the center of the kneecap. Press in while you lift and straighten your knee. You should feel this other very strong tendon, which is a long tendon common to both the two-joint quad and the one-joint quads.

The one-joint quads: These muscles begin on the front part of the "side and top of the thighbone." To find this beginning tendon, sit on a chair holding your hands a little below the "side and top of the thighbone." Press in here as you stand up, and you will feel the tendon move (another great place to massage). The muscle bellies extend down the outer side of the thigh and onto the knee. The ending tendon is the same as for the two-joint quad above.

To Feel the Muscles Move: Sit on a chair and, using both hands, grab the thigh of one leg. Position your hands so that you are pressing one thumb in the middle of the upper thigh and the other on the outer side, with your fingers wrapped around the bottom of the thigh. While pressing in, lift and straighten your knee, and feel the muscles moving (small movements make it easier to feel the muscle work).

Typical Traits

Understanding how and where this biggest and strongest muscle group in the body anchors to the bones, along with getting used to treating these sites, is the key to pain-free knees. All these muscles attach to one common tendon in which the kneecap is embedded. Therefore, it is no wonder that the kneecap can become affected in many ways by tension in these muscles. We use this muscle a lot because it is always active whenever the knee straightens—for example, during walking and climbing stairs. Since the muscle moves, stabilizes, and brakes the motion of the knee during jumping, lifting, running, sprinting, and deep squatting, it is the most stressed muscle group in such sports as volleyball, basketball, weight lifting, football, tennis, gymnastics, squash, high jump, long jump, and cycling. It provides an important braking action check. It reins the knee flexion on landing after jumping and functions as a shock absorber when running. When you lift a heavy load with bent knees, these muscles relieve much of the load from the lower back. (This is why lifting this way rather than with straight knees is recommended to prevent low back pain.) The quads are easy to strengthen by doing daily activities, but they seldom get a full stretch and are often unevenly strong, becoming more developed on one side. Knee problems due to imbalance of strength between the different quad muscles are very common. This can result in a pull on the patella, causing it to become misaligned. You abuse the quads during prolonged sitting because the fibers are then partially stretched for long hours, which can cause them to become weak. They respond to abuse by weakening.

Improvement Tip: Stand up and stretch your legs often if you sit a lot. Finding the tendons and treating them (circulation aid), stretching, and strengthening, depending on whether you are a sitter or physically active during your day.

Payoff: You can relieve yourself of pain in many different places on and around the knee if you take proper care of your quad muscles and their tendons. Making use of the bony landmarks to locate the tendon sites, massaging these sites regularly, and stretching the muscles can prove to be a surprisingly effective shortcut to pain relief for your knees.

The pain may be in front of the kneecap, just above it, on the side of the thigh while walking, or at the lower pole of the patella (jumper's knee—pain directly below the kneecap), which is one of the most common syndromes among athletes. You can relieve the patella of the pulling tension and misalignment caused by unevenly tight quads and weakness on knee straightening (buckling knee syndrome) by treating your quads. You can also stop pain from a patella that will not glide normally on the knee (locked patella syndrome), from adhesions and pain above the patella, and from inflammation of the patellar bursa. One quad, the rectus femoris, also bends the hip and develops syndromes of it own. Therefore, by stretching this muscle, you can help relieve hip and lower back problems due to a forward tilt of the hip bowl, as a tight rectus femoris can make it hard to fully straighten the hip.

Group
Opposing Muscles: In straightening the knee, the hamstrings, which bend the knee. In bending the hip, the gluteus maximus, which straightens the hip.

Assisting Muscles: In straightening the knee, the quads assist each other. In bending the hip, the iliopsoas, the tensor fasciae latae, and the adductors.

Muscles of the Foot

Bony Landmarks for the Muscles that Move the Foot

Many of these landmarks are the same as those for the muscles that move the knee. To find a few additional bony landmarks of the foot, trace your two lower leg bones down to your ankle with your fingers and you will notice a bump on each side right above your foot.

The outer bump of the ankle (external malleolus). This is the lower end of the fibula, the smaller and thinner outside bone of the lower leg.

The inner bump of the ankle (internal malleolus). This marks the end of the tibia, the large bone of the lower leg.

The heel bone (os calcis). This is the big round bone you can feel on the back of your heel.

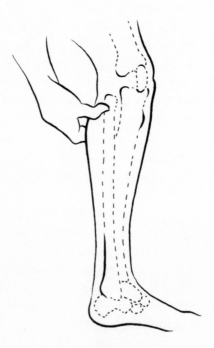

Foot

Bending the Foot Down—Pointing the Toes (Plantar Flexion)

The calf muscles include the two muscles in the back of the lower leg, one closer to the surface—the gastrocnemius, with two parts—and one deeper—

the soleus, with one part. The gastrocnemius, which we call the two-joint muscle here, has two parts and fits over two joints, the knee and the ankle. The soleus, the one-joint muscle, goes over the ankle only and not the knee. The two layers of calf muscles have different functions: the gastrocnemius plantar flexes, as in pointing the foot when the knee is straight, and the soleus plantar flexes the foot when the knee is bent. All three muscles join on the Achilles tendon.

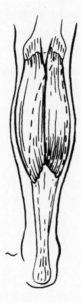

Calf muscles

Job

Bends the foot down, as in pointing the toes (plantar flexion).

Also:

Helps to bend the knee (flexion).
Helps to balance the body, preventing it from falling forward by contracting while the body is in a standing position.

How to Find It

To find the beginning tendons of the gastrocnemius, position your fingers on the back of your knee at the end of the thighbone (the thighbone ends at the knee, but is hard to locate in the back of the knee). One part begins on the "upper inside bump of the knee" in the back, and the other begins on the "upper outside bump of the knee" in the back. There are hamstring tendons here, making it difficult to get to the two gastrocnemius tendons. The one-joint calf muscle, which lies under the muscle just described, begins below the knee joint on the "lower inside bump of the knee" in the back. If you press in deep on the inner backside of your knee, right below the joint, you will be on this tendon.

To find the ending tendon, place your fingers on the back of your ankle a few inches above the heel and feel the thick Achilles tendon that stretches upward. This is the common ending tendon of the two calf muscles, and the thickest tendon in the body. If you pinch it, you will probably find that it is sore. Follow the tendon farther up the leg where it widens out into two muscle bellies.

To Feel the Muscle and Tendon Move: Place your fingers just under the back of your knee on the top of the calf and press in as you bend and straighten your foot. You can feel these muscles and tendons moving under your fingers. It takes experience to find the tendons behind your knee, because they are higher up than you might expect them to be.

Typical Traits

The calf muscles often seem just as difficult as the hamstrings to relax and relieve from stress. One reason for this is that only half of the calf muscles are stretched when you do calf stretches or engage in normal activities. Doing calf stretches with straight legs stretches only the outer layer of the muscles. The inner layer, which is usually more tense, gets no stretching. Bending the knees and then stretching, however, will stretch all the calf muscles. The calf muscles propel the body upward and forward while you run, jump, hop, bicycle, or dance on your toes; they push off the ground in walking, and balance your body when you stand. Running fast on hard surfaces or uphill puts these muscles under strain, as does wearing high-heeled shoes, which puts them in a contracted position. The muscle and tendon can also be vulnerable during twisting or during rotation movements. They tend to tighten when abused.

Improvement Tip: Stretching and circulation aid.

Payoff: Your calf muscles will feel more relaxed and comfortable, and you may experience fewer calf cramps at night. You may also relieve pain at the back of the knee and the instep of the foot, and leg cramps, which often develop when a person has been lying or sitting with the foot plantar flexed (pointed). To relieve sudden leg cramps at night, it helps to push the heel away from your body and bend your toes closer to the shinbone.

Group

Opposing Muscle: In bending the foot down and pointing the toes, the tibialis anterior, which bends the foot up.

Assisting Muscles: In bending the foot down and pointing the toes, the two calf muscles assist each other, and the peroneus also assists.

Bending the Foot Up (Dorsiflexion)

Tibialis anterior: Tibialis refers to the *shinbone,* and anterior means *front.*

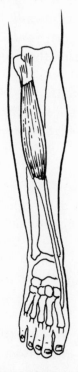

Tibialis anterior

Job

Bends the foot up (dorsal flexion).

Also:

> Helps to lift the inner ridge of the sole (inversion).
> Helps to maintain standing balance by contracting when the body sways too far backward.

How to Find It

To find the beginning tendon, sit with your knees bent. Place your thumb in the middle of the shinbone about an inch under the end of the kneecap, and reach around the outside of the leg with your fingers. Move your thumb an inch toward the outer side of the leg. Press in here, under the "lower outside bump of the knee," and you have found the tendon where it attaches to the sheath around the shinbone. Follow the muscle belly down the leg on the outer side of the shinbone. It narrows into a thick tendon that crosses over and ends on the inside of the foot. To find the ending tendon, place your foot on your knee, turning the sole up. Place your thumbs in the middle of the inside ridge of your foot, at the base of the big toe. Press in and feel the tightness here where the tendon attaches.

To Feel the Muscle and Tendon Move: While pressing in on and under the beginning tendon with your heel on the floor, lift your foot toward the shinbone, and feel the tendon bulge under your thumbs.

Typical Traits

This is the "shin splint" muscle and is very often the reason for pain in and under the big toe. Every time you lift your foot, you use it—for example, while walking, jogging, running, cycling, sprinting, and ice skating. It weakens with abuse.

Improvement Tip: Circulation aid at the tendon sites, strengthening, and stretching.

Payoff: By treating and strengthening this muscle, you may be able to heal and prevent intense pain in the front of the leg (shin splint) due to irritation of the sheath around the bone, right where this muscle's tendon attaches. The mysterious pain in your big toe and on the inside of the ankle may also disappear. If you strengthen and heal this muscle, your leg will get less tired when your lift to push a pedal or walk, you will be less prone to tripping due to weakness in this muscle, and it will no longer hurt when you squat with your heels on the floor.

Group

Opposing Muscle: In bending the foot up, the calf muscles, which bend the foot downward.

Assisting Muscles: In bending the foot up, the extensor digitorum longus. In lifting the inner ridge of the sole, the extensor hallucis longus.

Turning the Sole of the Foot out to the Side (Eversion)

The peroneus is a muscle with two parts that runs down the outer front of the lower leg, extending from the knee to the foot. Peroneus means *near the fibula.*

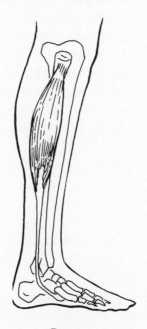

Peroneus

Job

Turns the sole of the foot out to the side (eversion).

Also:

Helps bend the foot down (plantar flexion).

How to Find It

To find the beginning tendon, place your fingers on the "lowest outside bump of the knee." Press and rub your fingers back and forth directly under this bone and you will feel the stringy beginning tendon. The belly stretches down the side of the lower leg to the ankle, and its tendon goes behind the outer anklebone, under a ligament, and then forward to the outside of the foot. From there, it crosses under the sole of the foot and ends on the base of the big toe bone on the opposite side of this bone as the tibialis anterior muscle. To find the ending tendon, press in on the back side of the outer anklebone while you turn the sole of your foot out to the side. The thick tendon bulges under your fingers.

To Feel the Muscle and Tendon Move: Turn your foot outward while pressing in on your lower leg, right under the beginning tendon, and you can feel the muscle moving under your fingers.

Nerve: The peroneal nerve can get trapped where it passes under the peroneal muscle right at its beginning attachment. You can sense the nerve if you press in really hard and rub the area of the beginning attachment. The tingling shoots down over the surface of the toes.

Typical Traits

This is the muscle that is susceptible to injury when you fall and twist your ankle so that your foot is suddenly inverted. You use this muscle, among others, when you walk, jog, and ice skate.

Improvement Tip: Circulation aid; thorough stretching and strengthening.

Payoff: You can improve the stability and strength of your ankles considerably by healing and strengthening this muscle. Strengthening can help prevent pain, weakness, and repeated sprains to the ankle after trauma has occurred; it can also protect your ankle from fractures caused by weak peroneus muscles.

Group

Opposing Muscle: In turning the sole of the foot out to the side, the tibialis anterior, which turns the inner ridge of the foot inward.

Assisting Muscle: In turning the sole of the foot out to the side, the extensor digitorum longus.

Lifting the Toes (Extension)

The extensor digitorum longus and extensor hallucis longus muscles lift the five toes. The extensor hallucis longus lifts the big toe only. Extensor means *stretch out,* and hallucis means *great toe.*

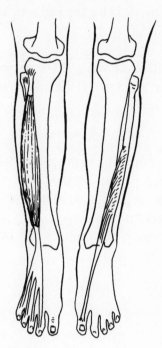

Extensor digitorum and extensor hallicus longus

Job

Lifts the big toe (hallucis longus).
Lifts the four other toes (digitorum).

Also:

Helps to bends the foot up (extension).
Helps to inverts the foot, lifting the inner ridge of the sole.

How to Find It

To find the beginning tendon, place your fingers on the "lower outside bump of the knee" and also on the "lowest outside bump of the knee." Lift your toes up, and feel the tendon here move slightly. The muscle belly extends down the lower leg and crosses over to go down into the big toe and the other toes. To find the beginning tendon of the hallucis longus, place your fingers on the "lowest outside bump of the knee" and follow this bone about one-third down the lower leg. Press in here while you lift your big toe only. It takes some practice to find this tendon. To find the ending tendon, lift your toes and big toe and watch the prominent tendons rise on the top of your foot.

To Feel the Muscle and Tendon Move: The muscle belly is hidden under other muscles, so the best place to feel the muscle move is at the beginning tendon site.

Typical Traits

Having feet that hurt is something many people take for granted, but such pain can be relieved when you understand how much the muscles of the feet contribute to it. A great way to avoid pain on the top of the foot and under the sole and to prevent night foot cramps is to maintain a balanced strength relationship between the muscles that lift (extend) the toes and those that bend (flex) them.

Group

Opposing Muscle: In lifting the big toe, the flexor hallucis longus (not a key muscle), which bends the big toe.

Assisting Muscle: In lifting the big toe, the extensor digitorum longus.

CHAPTER 10

Range of Motion

Recently I went to see a doctor. At the initial appointment, he measured the range of motion of my neck. He noticed that I was very restricted when turning my neck to the right side and asked me if I was aware of this, which I was not. After giving it some thought, however, I remembered that it had become harder and harder to see behind me when I was backing my car out of the garage. I had started twisting my body to get a full view. Except for this, which I had never really considered a problem, I had not noticed anything that indicated that my neck was not normal. I was quite surprised when the doctor informed me that I had severe restriction and deviation from the normal range of motion in my neck.

—Scott

We have not been taught to be aware of changes in flexibility and strength occurring over time due to our habits, lifestyles, and work conditions. This is, however, something that we can learn so we can detect muscle tightness early on and prevent future pain.

What Is Range of Motion?

Our joints have specific full ranges within which they function as long as the muscles are healthy. You can test these ranges by measuring the angle where the joint bends to its full extent. For example, when you bend your wrist, it will go only so far before it stops.

A SIMPLE RANGE OF MOTION TEST

Place your forearms on a table, palms facing each other. Bend the arm at the elbow, pointing your fingers toward the ceiling. Now bend your wrist, and you'll notice the angle that appears between your hand and the forearm bone, viewed from the thumb side. The degree of this angle is your range of motion for wrist flexion. Chapter 11 allows you to test your range to see if it is normal.

Physical therapists use a goniometer to measure the angle of the joint. This is a plastic device with two arms, one fixed and one moving, joined to form a corner with an adjustable angle.

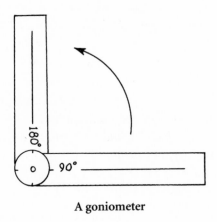

A goniometer

When you measure your own range, it helps you to approximate the degree of the standard range if you keep in mind simple angles such as an L-shaped right angle, 90 degrees, and half of that, 45 degrees.

Standard Range and Tests

When a physical therapist measures your range of motion, he compares your range to a standard range, measured in degrees, that has been developed over time by doctors and physical therapists. The standard is defined as the minimum range of motion a joint should have in order for the muscles to have a healthy function. This range indicates an optimum muscle length that allows for functional movement and for the joints to be properly aligned, which helps normal circulation of blood to the muscles and freedom from pain.

The Joints

It is not uncommon to be fearful of moving (the joints) to full range of motion because we are in doubt about how much motion they can tolerate. Shouldn't we protect them so they don't get damaged?

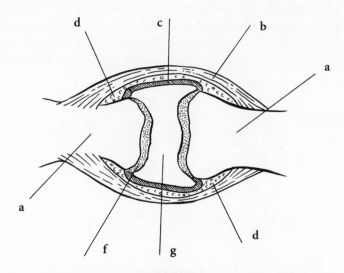

A synovial joint (a) bone; (b) ligament; (c) synovial membrane;
(d) bursa; (e) bone; (f) cartilage; (g) synovial fluid

The joints can indeed tolerate motion. This is why: Inside each of the main joints of your body (synovial joints) is a fluid-filled cavity that allows the bones to move in a fluid space, rather than grind on each other. This fluid, synovial fluid, brings nutrients to the joint and its protective pads (cartilage), and is produced inside the joint while you move. Your joints depend on the fluid for their health. Movement to full range of motion is therefore not only good for your joints, it is necessary.

Another reason why many people restrict their range of motion is that they don't quite know in what direction and how far they actually are safely able to move. Therefore, taking a look at the main joints in the body and how they function before you start measuring their ranges can be helpful.

The Joints of Your Neck (Cervical Spine)

When your head makes small rocking motions, as in nodding, you move a joint between the skull and the first vertebra (occipita-atlas) that consists of two small, bony sleds on the skull that fit and slide in two caved sockets on the first vertebra of the spine (C1). Half of all the forward- and backward-bending motion of the neck happens right here, while the other half relies on the joints between each of the six remaining neck vertebrae (C2–C7). These joints provide a flexibility that allows you to touch your chin to your chest when you bend your head forward and face the ceiling when you bend backward, as well as tilt your head to the side.

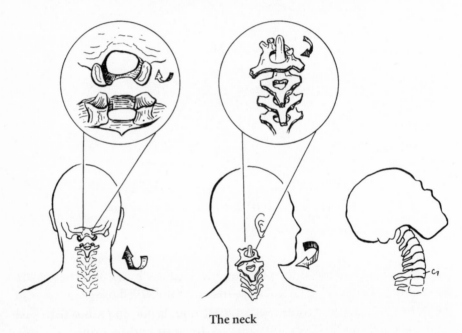

The neck

When you turn your head and look over your shoulder, you use a joint that is especially designed to rotate consisting of the two first verte-bra (C1, C2). The lower of the two (C2) has a bony prominence that the other (C1) pivots on, like a ring on a ring toss, allowing a wide turning range to both sides.

The Joints of Your Shoulder

The shoulder's vast mobility stems from the ball-and-socket structure of the big round top of the upper arm bone, which sits on a small, caved-in socket on the thin, flat shoulder blade (the glenohumeral joint). To make this unit stronger, the shoulder blade is wrapped on both sides in small muscles (the rotator cuff muscles) that reach over and attach to the upper arm bone.

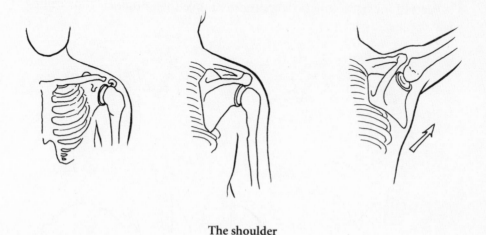

The shoulder

The purpose of the shoulder blades is to take the load off the shoulder joint as well as to provide a wider range of motion. It does this by gliding out to the side when the upper arm bone moves to full range in forward and sideways motions, thus adding to the range. When you move your arm backward, the range is more limited because the bottom corner of the shoulder blade swings down and in toward the center of the body and stops at the spine.

The purpose of the collarbone is to provide an attachment for the shoulder blades and tie the shoulder girdle together, which it does through a joint at the tip of the shoulder, called the "acromion process," where an extended part of the shoulder blade meets the collarbone.

The Joints of Your Upper and Lower Back
(Thoracic and Lumbar Spine)

The long column of vertebrae is flexible due to the soft pads (disks) that lie between them, allowing them to tip forward, backward, and sideways on the pads.

When you bend backward, a vertebra can tip only so far before it hits the bony part of another vertebra. Therefore, the back is not very mobile compared to, for example, the shoulder, the knee, or the elbow joint.

Parts of the back, however, are more mobile than others.

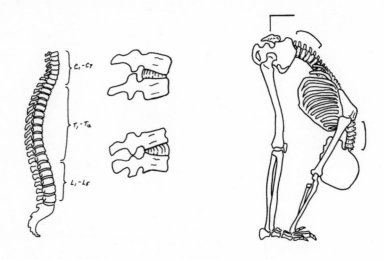

The back

The upper back is called the thoracic spine (T1–T12). These vertebrae are designed mainly to turn, or rotate. This is the least flexible part of the spine, and cannot bend forward, backward, or sideways very much.

The lower back is called the lumbar spine (L1–L5). These vertebrae are specifically designed to bend forward, backward, and sideways. This is the most flexible part of the spine.

When you bend forward to touch the floor with your hands, it seems as if your back moves to a large range of motion, but the back only bends for part (about half) of this range. Most of this bending movement (90 degrees) happens at the hip joint. For the ranges of the joints, see the next chapter.

The Joints of Your Hip and the Pelvic Girdle

The only real moving joint of the hip is at the bottom of each side of the hip bowl where the thighbones join the bowl. This is a ball-and-socket joint. The round top of the thighbone moves in a caved dent in the lower side of the hip bowl. The thighbone performs all the movements of the hip joint.

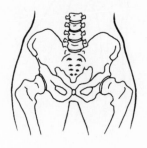
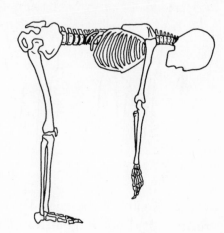

The hip

The hip bowl itself, the pelvic girdle, has its own motion. The hip bowl tilts forward (as it does if you are front-heavy and have weak stomach muscles), backward (as it does if you do not have good lower back support while sitting in a chair), to the side (as it does if one leg is shorter than the other), and into a tilt where one side is forward and the other side backward (as it can do if your hip flexors or extensors are unevenly tight), which is called an anterior/posterior tilt. Because the bowl and the spine joint are fused (sacrum), when the position of the hip bowl changes, it also changes the position of the spine and all the bones related to it. Whenever the bowl tilts, it pulls the spine with it.

The Joints of Your Knee

The knee joint is the largest joint in the body. When you bend the knee, the end of the thighbone (femur) moves on two indentations at the top of the lower leg bone (tibia) corresponding to the thighbone bumps.

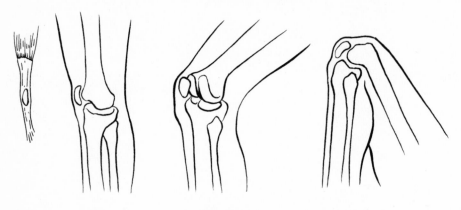

The knee

The stability of the knee depends totally on ligaments and muscle structures. It is not without reason that the front thigh muscles are the strongest muscle group in the body. The kneecap (patella) protects the knee joint. This bone is loose and not connected to other bones, but is held in place by the tendon of the front thigh muscles that extend over the knee to attach on the lower leg bone.

The Joints of Your Ankle

The foot is able to flip upward, with the toes toward the shin, and downward, with the toes toward the heel, because it is held by the lower leg bones like an object in a wrench. The ends of the largest leg bone (tibia) and the narrower one (fibula) grip around the foot bone (talus) at the ankle. These are the only motions the joint allows except for a slight rotation inside the wrench. With this limited range, how is it that we have a great ability to rotate the foot in circles? By a combined action of the wrench joint and two other joints between the bones in the center of the foot. These are not specifically ankle joints, but they allow the foot to invert and evert by giving it a good rotational capacity.

The Joints of Your Elbow

When you bend your elbow, the wide end of the forearm bone (ulna), which is shaped almost like a hook, glides around the upper arm bone. The joint is composed of three bones: the upper arm bone (humerus), the inner

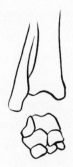

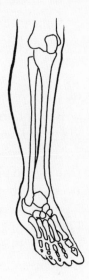

The ankle

forearm bone (radius), and the outer forearm bone (ulna). As in the knee, the upper arm bone widens out and ends in two bony bumps (medial and lateral epicondyles) at the elbow.

In addition to bending and straightening the arm, the bones of the elbow also rotate the hand. As long as the hand is palm-up, the two fore-arm bones are lying side by side in a parallel position. When you rotate the wrist so that the palm faces down, the inner forearm bone (radius), which is attached to the thumb side of the wrist, is pulled over the outer forearm bone at the wrist and crossed over it. When you move the wrist palm-up

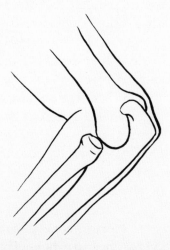

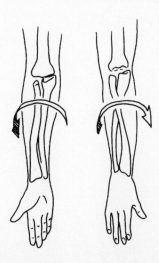

The elbow

again, the two bones are uncrossed. (It is not really the elbow joint that provides this motion, but rather a joint close to the elbow between the two lower arm bones.)

The Joints of Your Wrist

To find the wrist joint, follow the forearm bone starting on the inside of the elbow and going down the forearm to the thumb. You will feel how the bone widens out and extends toward the thumb, with one side ending in a bony bump (the styloid process of the radius) before the thumb. The wrist joints are between this bone and two rows of small, square wrist bones put together like puzzle pieces (the radiocarpal joint). The wrist and hand joints actually consist of 29 bones, but 19 of these belong to the fingers and extend into the hand. Eight small bones in the wrist, arranged in two rows, give the wrist and hand its fine-motor ability.

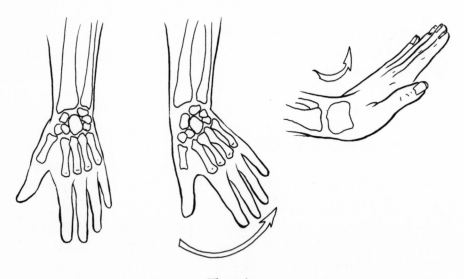

The wrist

The Joints of Your Fingers

The muscles that move the finger bones are very long and extend up the forearm to attach at the elbow. The fingers are therefore like puppets on a string, each having three bones held together by two joints. They can only bend or straighten, except for the bases of the fingers, which can spread (abduct) and move closer together (adduct).

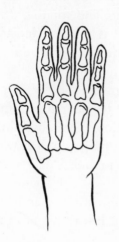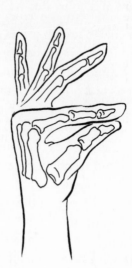

The fingers

The Joints of Your Thumb

The thumb differs from the fingers in that it has only two bones (excluding the bone in the hand). It also has an additional type of joint, a saddle joint, at the wrist, which permits the thumb to make many movements that the other fingers cannot do.

Testing

These home tests are designed so that you can get an approximate evalua-tion of the condition of your muscles and help you know where to work to improve their health and reduce pain. Although the measurements you will gather in the self-tests are not precise and therefore not clinically cor-rect, they can still provide you with very helpful information.

The different movements whose ranges you will be testing are the movements that your joints perform repetitively throughout the day, such as bending forward, bending backward, turning, and rotating different parts of your body. Each home test in this chapter is based on and adapted from tests that physical therapists use to determine range of motion. These tests measure the angles (in degrees) of the bending joint.

When you do the tests, the motions may seem ridiculously simple, yet it is in these everyday actions that the pattern for the pain in your muscles is found and where tightness and weakness develop. From observing how it feels to perform the tests (tight, painful, or natural), as well as what the range is, you can gain the information you need to understand your indi-vidual condition.

Through these simple motions, you can also explore and become familiar with how your joints function as well as learn what key muscles operate them.

What You Need

To perform the tests you will need a light, foot-long plastic ruler and a pen or a pencil. Some tests will require that you look in a mirror. Each test will guide you through the movement, describing how to estimate the range and mark your results. Be sure to repeat the test for both the left and right sides, if this applies.

You determine tightness in your muscles by measuring the range at the joint, notated by N for normal, T for tight, and TT for very tight. If you mark N, you know you are within the standard range.

Tools Provided

In the back of the book you will find:

• A chart on which to write down which muscles are tight. This chart can be a useful tool to refer to when your muscles start improving and you want to see where you started from.

• A blank pain chart on which to write down spots that are painful; this can help you start to see a pattern. Maybe they are all on one side of the body. Maybe they cross from one side to the other. These will change as you work on stretching and strengthening, and it is a great feeling when you notice that you no longer have pain in spots that used to hurt.

Interpreting Your Results

If you marked *T* or *TT* in the range test, the next step is to find out which muscle is causing the problem and how.

The most likely muscle to cause restricted range while bending in one direction is the muscle that bends in the opposite direction. For example, if you are restricted in bending the head (ear to shoulder) to one side, you look for tightness in the muscle that bends the head to the other side.

Note: Muscles work in pairs of opposites. The primary mover performs the action, while the opposing muscle has to stretch and relax to allow this action to take place (see Chapter 4 about muscle groups and balance). Therefore, if the range is limited, we look for tightness in the opposing muscle.

The next likely muscle to cause restricted range while bending in one direction, if the opposing muscle is not the culprit, is the primary mover. For example, if you cannot bend your trunk backward to full range and the abdominal muscles are not tight, you look to the back muscles. Are they too pained, tight, or weak to contract adequately? Weakness in the primary mover is not very often the reason for restricted range, but pain and tightness that make it hard to contract often are. Here we call this impaired function.

The "Interpreting Your Results" section that follows each test will identify these muscles and refer you first to the appropriate test for tightness in the opposing muscle. Next, you will be referred to the appropriate test for the primary mover.

Testing for tightness involves stretching the muscle slowly while observing if it hurts or the muscle noticeably resists stretching. Look up the muscle in the index, which will refer you to the page number for the right stretch. From the starting position, do the passive stretch very slowly and observe how the muscle works, hold, then relax. Is there pain or tension? Does the tension continue to increase the longer you hold the stretch, or does it release?

Your muscle should stretch evenly, without pain, and should notice-ably release when you hold the stretch.

Testing for impaired function in this book involves:

1. Observing the muscle as it contracts during a strengthening exer-cise to see if it loses power, tremors, and/or contracts unevenly. Again, look up the name of the muscle in the index, which will refer you to the right strength test.

2. Touching and palpating the muscle belly and tendon sites as you perform the test. The index will refer you to the page that describes how to locate the muscle belly and its tendon sites.

Do one or two strengthening exercises and observe the muscle. The tests provided for each muscle are meant to help you determine if you have the minimum strength necessary for basic function of the muscle.

What to Do with the Information You Collect

Chapter 5 tells you what steps to take to heal, stretch, and strengthen your muscle back to health.

Before beginning any of the tests, it is important to assume the starting position (see Chapter 4). This correctly aligned posture will make sure that your joints are in a position to safely handle any movement, whether bending, turning, or stretching. It also allows you to breathe more easily, which provides more oxygenated blood to the muscles, enabling them to go into the range better.

CHAPTER 11

Testing Your Key Muscles

You can learn to recognize tightness and pain levels in your key muscles. You do this by testing the range of flexibility of the joints these muscles operate (range of motion testing); for example, how far your arm can extend out to the side and up, or how far your back can bend. The tests refer you to stretches, strengthening exercises, and self-treatment for the muscles involved.

As you perform these home tests, you'll become familiar with what key muscles (hamstrings, triceps, calf muscles, etc.) are responsible for your everyday movements, which helps you to spot problems in your muscles before pain develops.

To facilitate marking test results, spaces are provided following questions within this chapter, but you may also record test results in the chart on pages 271–272 if you'd like to have a complete log.

Neck Tests

Home Test 1: Bending Forward (Flexion)

Primary Mover: Sternocleidomastoid (SCM)
Opposing Muscles: Splenius capitis, splenius cervicis

From the starting position, sitting or standing, slowly bend your head toward your chest, releasing the head first and then the neck, vertebra by vertebra. Do not force the movement, and let the neck bend only as far as it will go comfortably. Keep your shoulders and upper back immobile. Do not (a) hold the head too far forward or back (your ears should be over your shoulders), (b) bend your upper body forward, (c) roll your shoulders forward, or (d) open your mouth.

When you cannot bend forward any farther, record the following information:

If you can fit one finger knuckle under your chin ($3/4''$ or less), mark N. _____

If you can fit two to three finger knuckles under your chin,
mark T.   _____

If you can fit your whole fist under your chin (place the fist
on your chest, little finger down, where the collarbones
come together in front), mark TT.   _____

If it hurts on both sides of the spine, mark L/R.   _____

If it hurts more on one side than the other, mark L or R.   _____

If there is no pain, mark N.   _____

Interpreting Your Results

If the range is *TT* or *T*: first, test the *opposing muscles* for *tightness:* the splenius capitis and the splenius cervicis, which bend the neck backward (slow stretch). Next, test the *primary movers:* the SCM muscles, which bend the neck forward (impaired function test). Note: Gravity helps to pull the head down, so weakness does not limit this motion much.

If the range is *N* but your muscles still ache, turn to Chapter 5, "Starting the Healing Process."

Standard Range: The head/neck is able to bend 45 degrees forward.

Home Test 2: Bending Backward (Extension)

Primary Movers: Splenius capitis, splenius cervicis
Opposing Muscles: SCMs, scalenes

Stand by a mirror so you can check your profile. Choose a spot on the ceiling right above your head as a reference point. For this test, it is helpful if you can hold the end of a light plastic ruler in your mouth, but you can also use your nose as a guide to measuring the angle. From the starting position, bend your head/neck backward in small increments as far as it will go. (While looking in the mirror, you may discover interesting errors in perception—you may feel as if you have bent your head 90 degrees backward when in reality it is only 45 degrees at the most.) Do not (a) stay extended too long—it alarms the tension/length monitors in addition to squeezing your vertebrae's disks, (b) move your trunk or shoulders, or (c) roll your eyes instead of your head. *Note:* gravity helps to pull the head backward, so this movement is not limited much by weakness.

When your head can't go back any farther record the following information:

If the ruler or your nose points almost straight up to the
    ceiling spot, mark N.   _____

If it points ¾ of the way up, mark T.   _____

If it stops halfway between the starting point and the
    ceiling spot, mark TT.   _____

If it hurts on both sides of the spine, mark L/R.   _____

If it hurts more on one side, mark L or R.   _____

If it does not hurt, mark N.   _____

Interpreting Your Results

If the range is *TT* or *T:* first, test the opposing muscles for tightness, the
scalenes and the SCMs, which bend the neck forward (slow stretch). Next,
test the primary movers, the splenius capitis and splenius cervicis muscles,
which bend the neck backward (impaired function test).

If the range is *N* but your muscles still ache, turn to Chapter 5,
"Starting the Healing Process."

Standard Range: The neck is able to bend 45 degrees backward, with the
face almost, but not quite, flat toward the ceiling.

Home Test 3: Turning and Rotating the Head and Neck (as in Looking over Your Shoulder; lateral rotation)

Primary Mover: SCM on the opposite side of the direction the face is
being turned toward
Opposing Muscle: SCM on the same side that the face is being turned
toward

Stand in the starting position, sideways to a mirror so you can check your
profile. Slowly rotate your head toward the mirror. Watch your head closely as you turn it. You will probably notice that what feels like a 90-degree
turn is really only 75 degrees at the most. Do not (a) turn your upper body
or shoulders, (b) tilt your head backward or forward, (c) tilt your head to
the side, or (d) move your shoulders.

Note: You can also do this test by lying on the floor with the end of a
ruler in your mouth. Turn your head to one side and estimate the distance
from the floor to the ruler, and then repeat to the other side.

When your head is fully turned to one side, record the following
information:

If your nose (or ruler) stops about three-quarters of the way
  or farther from the starting position to the side, mark N.   _____
If your nose points a little farther than halfway, mark T.   _____
If your nose points halfway between 90 degrees and the
  starting point, mark TT.   _____

Repeat with the other side and compare the results.

If you have pain on both sides, mark L/R.   _____
If it hurts more on one side than on the other, mark L or R.   _____
If you have no pain, mark N.   _____

Interpreting Your Results

If the range is *TT* or *T*: first, test the opposing muscles for tightness, the SCM on the same side, which rotates the head to the opposite side and resists turning to the same side (slow stretch). Next, test the primary mover, the SCM on the opposite side, which rotates the neck to the opposite side (impaired function test).

If the range is *N* but your muscles still ache, turn to Chapter 5, "Starting the Healing Process".

Standard Range: The neck is able to turn 75 degrees to the side.

Home Test 4: Bending Sideways (Lateral Flexion)
Primary Mover: Scalene on same side
Opposing Muscle: Scalene on opposite side

Stand in the starting position facing a mirror. Make sure your head is not tilted to either side (your chin should be over the point where the collarbones meet). Place a ruler horizontally in your mouth, biting on the six-inch mark (middle). Slowly tilt your head to the side, bringing your ear toward your shoulder. Keep your shoulders still and let the vertebrae release one by one. Do not (a) lift one shoulder, (b) lift one side of your torso, or (c) rotate your head/torso to one side.

Looking at where the end of the ruler stops, record the following information:

If the ruler stops an inch or two below the tip of the shoulder,
  mark N.   _____
If the ruler stops right at the tip of the shoulder, mark T.   _____

If it stops one or two inches in the air above the shoulder,
　　mark TT.   _____

Repeat the test for the other side and compare the results.

　　If it hurts on both sides, mark L/R.   _____
　　If it hurts more on one side than on the other, mark L or R.   _____
　　If there is no pain, mark N.   _____

Interpreting Your Results

If the range is *TT* or *T:* first, test the opposing muscles for tightness, the
scalenes on the opposite side, which bend the neck to their side (slow
stretch). Next, test the primary movers, the scalenes on the same side,
which bend the neck to the same side (impaired function test).

　　If the range is *N* but your muscles still ache, turn to Chapter 5,
"Starting the Healing Process."

Standard Range: The neck is able to bend 45 to 60 degrees to the side.

Shoulder Tests

Home Test 1: Shrugging the Shoulders (Elevation)
Primary Movers: Upper trapezius, levator scapulae, rhomboids
Opposing Muscles: Lower trapezius, latissimus dorsi, serratus anterior

Stand in front of a mirror in the starting position. Look at your shoulders.
Are they level on both sides when you stand relaxed? Pay attention to
where the collarbones meet in front over the breastbone. (Follow the collarbones from the shoulders toward the center.) Are these two points even?
Now, slowly shrug your shoulders up toward your ears. In this position,
record the following information:

　　If both shoulders go equally high, mark =   _____
　　If it hurts on both sides, mark L/R.   _____
　　If it hurt more on one side than on the other, mark L or R.   _____
　　If there is no pain, mark N.   _____

Interpreting Your Results
If the range is TT or T: first, test the opposing muscles, the lower trapezius, the latissimus dorsi, and the serratus anterior, which depress the

shoulder (slow stretch). Next, test the primary movers, the upper trapezius, the levator scapulae, and the rhomboids, which raise the shoulder (impaired function test).

If the range is N but your muscles still ache, turn to Chapter 5, "Starting the Healing Process."

Standard Range: Shrugging the shoulders is not a "pure" joint movement. Therefore, there is no standard range that we can compare ourselves to; however, the shoulders should be able to rise up almost to your ears.

Home Test 2: Raising the Arms up in Front of the Body (Shoulder Flexion)

Primary Movers: Deltoid (front part), pectoralis major
Opposing Muscles: Deltoid (back part), teres major, triceps (long part), latissimus dorsi

Lie on the floor with both knees bent, your feet flat on the floor, and both hip bones on the floor. Do not (a) let your lower back arch more than a little, (b) bend your elbows, or (c) let your arms move out to the side. Hold your arms with your palms down and your elbows straight. Slowly raise your arms up toward the ceiling and back as far as you can, aiming to rest your arms on the floor above your head.

In this position, record the following information for each arm:

If your arm goes comfortably all the way to the floor, mark N. _____

If your arm stops a couple of inches above the floor, mark T.   _____
If your arm stops 10 inches or more above the floor, mark TT. _____

Compare sides:

If both sides hurt, mark L/R.   _____
If one side hurts more than the other, mark L or R.   _____
If there is no pain, mark N.   _____

Interpreting Your Results

If the range is *TT* or *T*: first, test the opposing muscles for tightness, the back part of the deltoid, the teres major, the long part of the triceps, and the latissimus dorsi, which all lift the arm up behind the body (slow stretch).

Next, test the primary movers, the front part of the deltoid and the pectoralis major, which lift the arm up in front of the body (impaired function test).

If the range is N but your muscles still ache, turn to Chapter 5, "Starting the Healing Process."

Standard Range: The shoulders allow bending of the arm at the shoulder to 180 degrees (straight above the head).

Home Test 3: Raising the Arm up behind the Body (Shoulder Extension)
Primary Movers: Deltoid (back part), latissimus dorsi
Opposing Muscle: Deltoid (front part)

Stand in the starting position with your elbow bent to 90 degrees and held close to the hip. Do not (a) lift or rotate your shoulders, (b) bend your upper back forward, or (c) hold your elbows out to the side. Notice where your wrist is positioned (your palm is facing toward your body) as you move your elbow backward as far as it goes.

In this position, record the following information for each arm:

If your wrist moves all the way to ribs and farther, mark N.   _____
If it moves almost to the ribs, mark T.   _____
If your wrist moves halfway to the ribs, mark TT.   _____

Compare sides:

If it hurts on both sides, mark L/R.   _____
If it hurts more on one side than on the other, mark L or R.   _____
If there is no pain, mark N.   _____

Interpreting Your Results
If the range is TT or T: first, test the opposing muscle for tightness, the front part of the deltoid, which lifts the arm up in front of the body (slow stretch). Next, test the primary movers, the back part of the deltoid and the latissimus dorsi, which lift the arm up in back of the body (impaired function test).

If the range is N but your muscles still ache, turn to Chapter 5, "Starting the Healing Process."

Standard Range: The arms (shoulders) are able to move backward about 50 degrees.

Home Test 4: Raising the Arm up to the Side (Abduction of Shoulder Joint)

Primary Movers: Deltoid (middle part), supraspinatus
Opposing Muscles: Pectoralis major, latissimus dorsi

Lie on the floor with your knees bent, feet flat on the floor, and hipbones on the floor. Do not (a) bend your trunk, (b) bend the elbows, or (c) hold the hands palms-down. Keep your elbows straight and turn your hands palms-up. Move your arms out to the side as far as they will go toward your ears.

In this position, record the information for each arm:

If your arm goes up so your arms contact the side of
your head, mark N.   _____

If your arm stops a few inches away from your head,
mark T.   _____

If your arm goes only halfway between 90 degrees
(to the side) and straight up, mark TT.   _____

Compare sides:

If it hurts on both sides, mark L/R.   _____
If it hurts more on one side than on the other, mark L or R.   _____
If there is no pain, mark N.   _____

Interpreting Your Results

If the range is *TT* or *T*: first, test the opposing muscles for tightness, the pectoralis major and the latissimus dorsi, which move the shoulder in toward the body (slow stretch).

Next, test the primary movers, the middle part of the deltoid and the supraspinatus (not a key muscle), which move the shoulder out to the side and up (impaired function test).

If the range is *N* but your muscles still ache, turn to Chapter 5, "Starting the Healing Process."

Standard Range: The shoulders allow the arms to move out 180 degrees (to the ears).

Home Test 5: Pulling the Arm down to the Side (Adduction of Shoulder Joint)

Primary Movers: Pectoralis major, latissimus dorsi
Opposing Muscles: Deltoid (middle part), supraspinatus

Lie on the floor, same as above, with the arms out to the side (150 degrees). Bring your arms in toward your body. Do not hold your hands palms-up. Pay attention to how willing the arm is to move all the way in. Do your shoulders feel tight when the arms are held in to the side? Record the following information for each arm:

> If your arm goes comfortably all the way in, mark N.   _____
> If you have to force your arms to stay in toward the body,
>   mark T.   _____
> If your arm stops a few inches or more away from the body,
>   mark TT.   _____

Compare sides:

> If it hurts on both sides, mark L/R.   _____
> If it hurts more on one side than on the other, mark L or R.   _____
> If there is no pain, mark N.   _____

Interpreting Your Results

If the range is *TT* or *T:* first, test the opposing muscles for tightness, the middle part of the deltoid (slow stretch) and the supraspinatus (not a key muscle), which move the shoulder up and out to the side. Next, test the primary movers, the pectoralis major (impaired function test) and the latissimus dorsi, which move the shoulder in toward the body.

   If the range is *N* but your muscles still ache, turn to Chapter 5, "Starting the Healing Process."

Standard Range: The shoulders allow the arms to move in next to the trunk.

Home Test 6: Hugging Yourself (Horizontal Adduction)

Primary Movers: Pectoralis major (upper part), deltoid (front part)
Opposing Muscles: Deltoid (back part), pectoralis major (lower part)

Stand or sit in the starting position. Hold your arms in front of you, palms-down, and bend your arms at the elbow to 90 degrees (as if placing your hands on a flat surface in front of you). Slowly move both bent elbows across the front of your chest, crossing one elbow and forearm over the other. Alternate upper and lower to see if both are equally able to move across the chest.

Record the following information, noting any difference in range between the side:

> If you can cross your elbows over and past each other,
> mark N.   _____
> If your elbows do not quite meet, mark T.   _____
> If your elbows stop eight or more inches away from each
> other, mark TT.   _____
> If it hurts on both sides, mark L/R.   _____
> If it hurts more on one side than on the other, mark L or R.   _____
> If there is no pain, mark N.   _____

Interpreting Your Results

If the range is *TT* or *T*: first, test the opposing muscles for tightness, the back part of the deltoid and the infraspinatus, which move the shoulder out to the side and back (slow stretch).

Next, test the primary movers, the pectoralis major and the front part of the deltoid, which move the shoulder and arm across the chest (impaired function test).

If the range is *N* but your muscles still ache, turn to Chapter 5, "Starting the Healing Process."

Standard Range: The shoulder blades can move 120 degrees in this direction (90 degrees of this is left hand on the right elbow and right hand on the left elbow, plus 30 degrees across the chest).

Home Test 7: Raising the Arms Straight out Front and Moving Them toward the Back (Horizontal Abduction of the Shoulder)

Primary Movers: Deltoid (back part), infraspinatus
Opposing Muscles: Pectoralis major, deltoid (front part)

Stand in a doorway. Lift an arm straight out forward, perpendicular to the floor, and bend the elbow to 90 degrees, moving the forearm across your chest. Move your elbow to the side (straight out from the shoulder, elbow pointing to the door frame). Check that the hip and the shoulder/elbow are in line with the length of the door frame. Do not turn your trunk or hips. Keep your body steady and watch your wrist move in relation to the door frame when you pull your elbow backward. When it stops, notice where the wrist is located and record the following information for each side:

If your wrist is in the place your elbow was when you
    started, mark N.   _____
If your wrist stops right before the doorframe, mark T.   _____
If your wrist barely moves backward, mark TT.   _____

Compare sides:

If it hurts on both sides, mark L/R.   _____
If it hurts more on one side, mark L or R.   _____
If there is no pain, mark N.   _____

Interpreting Your Results

If the range is *TT* or *T:* first, test the opposing muscles for tightness, the pectoralis major, and the front part of the deltoid, which move the raised arms forward.

Next, test the primary movers, the back part of the deltoid and the infraspinatus, which move the arm backward.

If the range is *N* but your muscles still ache, turn to Chapter 5, "Starting the Healing Process."

Standard Range: The shoulder is able to move backward 40 degrees (from 90 degrees, which is arms straight out to the side).

Home Test 8: Hands-Up Position
(External Rotation of the Shoulder Joint)

Primary Movers: Deltoid (back part), infraspinatus
Opposing Muscles: Pectoralis major, subscapularis

Lie on the floor with your arms out to the side. Bend your elbows 90 degrees and point your fingers up toward the ceiling, palms facing your feet. Move your forearms back and down to the floor so that the back of your hand attempts to touch the floor. In this position, record the following information for each arm:

> If your arms rest comfortably on the floor, mark N.   _____
> If your arms do not rest comfortably on the floor, mark T.   _____
> If your arms do not reach the floor at all, mark TT.   _____

Compare sides:

> If it hurts on both sides, mark L/R.   _____
> If it hurts more on one side than on the other, mark L or R.   _____
> If there is no pain, mark N.   _____

Interpreting Your Results

If the range is *TT* or *T*: first, test the opposing muscles for tightness, the pectoralis major and the subscapularis (see appendix), which move the arm to a hands-down position (slow stretch).

Next, test the primary movers, the back part of the deltoid and the infraspinatus, which move the arm to a "hands-up" position (impaired function test).

If the range is *N* but your muscles still ache, turn to Chapter 5, "Starting the Healing Process."

Standard Range: 90 degrees.

Home Test 9: Rolled-In Shoulders
(Internal Rotation of the Shoulder Joint)

Primary Movers: Subscapularis, pectoralis major
Opposing Muscles: Infraspinatus, deltoid (back part)

Lie on the floor in the same starting position as above, with elbows bent and fingers pointing to the ceiling, palms facing your feet. Move your forearms and palms down to the floor in the direction of your feet, making sure that your shoulders do not lift off the floor. In this position, record the following information for each side:

> If your palms go down so they are 5 to 6 inches from the floor,
>   mark N.   _____
> If your forearms stop 15 inches from the floor, mark T.   _____
> If your forearms stop halfway between straight up and the
>   floor, mark TT.   _____

Compare sides:

If it hurts on both sides, mark L/R.   _____
If it hurts more on one side than on the other, mark
    L or R.   _____
If there is no pain, mark *N*.   _____

Interpreting Your Results

If the range is *TT* or *T*: first, test the opposing muscles for tightness, the infraspinatus (see appendix) and the back part of the deltoid, which move the arm to a hands-up position (slow stretch).

Next, test the primary movers, the subscapularis and the pectoralis major, which move the arm to a hands-down position (impaired function text).

If the range is *N* but your muscles still ache, turn to Chapter 5, "Starting the Healing Process."

Standard Range: 65 to 90 degrees.

Elbow Tests

Home Test 1: Bending the Elbow (Flexion)
Primary Movers: Biceps, brachioradialis
Opposing Muscle: Triceps

Sit on a chair with your arms hanging down by your sides, palms facing forward. Do not (a) move your arm forward at the shoulder or (b) hold your hands other than palms up. Keeping your elbow steady at your side, slowly bend your arm at the elbow and lift your forearm as far as it goes toward the shoulder. (The size of the biceps is a factor in how close to the upper arm the forearm can get.) Repeat with the other side, and record the following information for each side:

If you can touch your shoulder with your fingertips (you
    can bend your wrist), mark N.   _____
If your fingertips stop one inch away from the shoulder,
    mark T.   _____
If your arm stops halfway between 90 degrees and your
    shoulder, mark TT.   _____

Compare sides:

If it hurts on both sides, mark L/R.   _____

If it hurts more on one side than on the other, mark L or R.   _____

If there is no pain, mark N.   _____

Interpreting Your Results

If the range is *TT* or *T:* first, test the opposing muscles for tightness, the triceps, which straighten the elbow (slow stretch).

Next, test the primary movers, the biceps (see appendix) and the brachioradialis, which bend the arm at the elbow (impaired function test).

If the range is *N* but your muscles still ache, turn to Chapter 5, "Starting the Healing Process."

Standard Range: The elbow can bend to 145 degrees (90 plus 55).

Home Test 2: Straightening the Elbow (Extension)
Primary Mover: Triceps
Opposing Muscles: Biceps, brachioradialis

Stand sideways to a mirror with the arm facing the mirror bent at the elbow and the palm facing your body. Do not (a) bend (flex) your arm forward at the shoulder or (b) face your palms away from your body. Straighten the arm. Look in the mirror, and record the following information for each arm:

If your arm is straight and centered with the middle of the
   thigh, mark N.   _____
If your elbow is just a little bent, mark T.   _____
If your elbow is bent so the forearm is angled forward of
   the thigh, mark TT.   _____

Compare sides:
   If it hurts on both sides, mark L/R.   _____
   If it hurts more on one side than the other, mark L or R.   _____
   If there is no pain, mark N.   _____

Interpreting Your Results

If the range is *TT* or *T:* first, test the opposing muscles for tightness, the biceps (not a key muscle) and brachioradialis (slow stretch), which bend the arm at the elbow.

Next, test the primary movers, the triceps, which straighten the elbow (impaired function test).

If the range is *N* but your muscles still ache, turn to Chapter 5, "Starting the Healing Process."

Standard Range: The elbow can straighten to 145 degrees (not 180, because it does not start from a straight-up position).

Home Test 3: Turning the Forearm Palms Down (Pronation)

Primary Movers: Pronator teres, pronator quadratus
Opposing Muscle: Supinator

Sit facing a table so that you can place your forearms on the table with the palms facing each other and the hands pointing forward. Keeping your elbows by your sides and bent at a 90-degree angle, turn one of your forearms palm down (in toward the thumb side). Do not (a) move your elbows away from your body or (b) bend them more or less than 90 degrees. Repeat with the other arm.

Mark your results for each arm:

If your hand lies flat on the table, mark N.   _____

If your hand does not turn all the way down so the
    thumb is off the table, mark T.   _____

If your palms are making an angle with the table,
    mark TT.   _____

Compare sides:

If it hurts on both sides, mark L/R.   _____

If it hurts more on one side, mark L or R.   _____

If there is no discomfort, mark N.   _____

Interpreting Your Results

If the range is *T:* first, test the opposing muscle for tightness, the supinator, which rotates the forearm palms up (slow stretch).

Next, test the primary movers, the pronator teres (impaired function test) and the pronator quadratus (not a key muscle), which rotate the forearm palms down (impaired function test).

If the range is *N* but your muscles still ache, turn to Chapter 5, "Starting the Healing Process."

Standard Range: The elbow can rotate 90 degrees inward (with the palm all the way down).

Home Test 4: Turning the Forearm Palm Up (Supination)
Primary Mover: Supinator
Opposing Muscle: Pronator teres

Sit facing a table and place your forearms on the table with the palms facing each other. Do not (a) move your elbows away from your body or (b) bend them more or less than 90 degrees. Bend your elbows at 90 degrees and keep them by your sides. Turn your forearms palms up.
    Record the following information for each side:

If your hand rotates all the way over but the thumb side
    is slightly raised, mark N.   _____
If only the back of your hand at the little finger side
    touches the table, mark T.   _____
If no part of the back of your hand lies on the table,
    mark TT.   _____

Compare sides:

If it hurts on both sides, mark L/R.   _____
If it hurts more on one side, mark L or R.   _____
If there is no pain, mark N.   _____

Interpreting Your Results
If the range is *T* or *TT:* first, test the opposing muscle for tightness, the pronator teres, which rotates the forearm palms down (slow stretch).
    Next, test the primary mover, the supinator, which rotates the forearm palms up (impaired function test).
    If the range is *N* but your muscles still ache, turn to Chapter 5, "Starting the Healing Process."

Standard Range: The forearm can rotate to 90 degrees outward. However, it is normal to feel more comfortable to pronate (palms down) rather than supinate (palms up). We are simply more used to it.

Hand and Wrist Tests

Home Test 1: Bending the Hand (Flexion)

Primary Movers: Flexor carpi radialis, flexor carpi ulnaris, flexor digitorum, palmaris longus

Opposing Muscles: Extensor carpi radialis, extensor carpi ulnaris, extensor digitorum

Support your elbow on a table. Bend your arm at the elbow, keeping straight wrists, with your fingers pointing to the ceiling. Turn your palms so they face each other. Bend the hand so that you make an L shape at the wrist. Do not (a) turn your hand palm forward or (b) rotate the hand. Imagine a line between the knuckle at the base of the index finger and the back of the bent wrist on the thumb side. Notice the angle formed here. Repeat with the other wrist.

Record the following information for each hand:

If the wrist bends to an L-shaped (90-degree) angle,
    mark N.   _____

If the angle of your wrist is smaller than what you would
    estimate the midposition of your wrist to be (between
    straight up and an L shape,) mark T.   _____

If the angle is larger than it is at the midposition, mark TT.   _____

Compare sides:

If it hurts on both sides, mark L/R.   _____
If it hurts more on one side, mark L or R.   _____
If there is no pain, mark N.   _____

Interpreting Your Results

If the range is *T* to *TT:* first, test the opposing muscles for tightness, the extensor carpi radialis, the extensor carpi ulnaris, and the extensor digitorum, which move the wrist backward (slow stretch).

Next, test the primary movers, the flexor carpi radialis (impaired function test), the flexor carpi ulnaris, the flexor digitorum, and the palmaris longus, which bend the wrist forward (impaired function test).

If the range is *N* but your muscles still ache, turn to Chapter 5, "Starting the Healing Process."

Standard Range: The wrist can bend from 90 degrees.

Home Test 2: Lifting the Hand (Extension)
Primary Movers: Extensor carpi radialis, extensor carpi ulnaris, extensor digitorum
Opposing Muscles: Flexor carpi radialis, flexor carpi ulnaris, flexor digitorum, palmaris longus

Support your elbow on a table. Bend your arm at the elbow, keeping your wrist straight, with your fingers pointing to the ceiling. Turn your palms so they face each other. Bend the wrist backward (you can relax the fingers) and examine the angle formed by the back of your hand and the forearm bone, imagining a line running between the knuckle at the base of the index finger and the base of the thumb. Do not (a) rotate your hand or (b) tense your fingers. Repeat with the other wrist.

Mark the range for each side:

Estimate an angle of the wrist midway between holding it
   straight up and in a perfect L shape.
If your wrist moves well past this midway line, mark N.   _____
If it makes the 45-degree angle (midway), mark T.   _____
If it makes an angle less than 45 degrees, mark TT.   _____

Compare sides:

If it hurts on both sides, mark L/R.   _____
If it hurts more on one side, mark L or R.   _____
If there is no pain, mark N.   _____

Interpreting Your Results
If the range is *T* or *TT*: first, test the opposing muscles for tightness, the flexor carpi radialis, the flexor carpi ulnaris, the flexor digitorum, and the palmaris longus, which bend the wrist forward (slow stretch).

Next, test the primary movers, the extensor carpi radialis (impaired function test), the extensor carpi ulnaris, and the extensor digitorum, which lift the wrist backward (impaired function test).

If the range is *N* but your muscles still ache, turn to Chapter 5, "Starting the Healing Process."

Standard Range: The wrist is able to bend 70 degrees backward.

Home Test 3: Bending the Hand Sideways
toward the Little Finger Side (Ulnar Deviation)
Primary Movers: Flexor carpi ulnaris, extensor carpi ulnaris
Opposing Muscles: Flexor carpi radialis, extensor carpi radialis

Sit at a square-edged table. Mark a line in a perfect L shape right in front of you on the table. Place your hands palms down, your wrists at the edge of the table. Hold your elbows bent at 90 degrees. Line up your middle finger with the straight line of the L. Make sure an imaginary straight line runs through the mid-forearm and the middle finger. Then slide your wrist sideways toward the little finger side, keeping your forearm immobile. Do not (a) bend or extend your hand/wrist up or down or (b) move the forearm (only the wrist). Now imagine a line running between the knuckle at the base of your middle finger and the middle of your wrist as it moves away from the line on the table. Repeat with the other wrist.
    Mark the range for each wrist:

If this line moves past the midline between the two arms
    of the H shape, mark N.   _____
If it moves halfway or a little less, mark T.   _____
If it barely moves, mark TT.   _____

Compare sides:

If it hurts on both sides, mark L/R.   _____
If it hurts more on one side, mark L or R.   _____
If there is no pain, mark N.   _____

Interpreting Your Results
If the range is *T* or *TT*: first, test the opposing muscles for tightness, the flexor carpi radialis and the extensor carpi radialis, which move the hand toward the thumb side (slow stretch).
    Next, test the primary movers, the flexor carpi ulnaris (impaired function test) and the extensor carpi ulnaris, which move the hand toward the little-finger side (impaired function test).

If the range is *N* but your muscles still ache, turn to Chapter 5, "Starting the Healing Process."

Standard Range: The wrist can bend 35 degrees to the little finger side.

Home Test 4: Bending the Hand Sideways toward the Thumb Side (Radial Deviation)

Primary Movers: Flexor carpi radialis, extensor carpi radialis
Opposing Muscles: Flexor carpi ulnaris, extensor carpi ulnaris

Sit at a square-edged table. Mark a line in a perfect L shape in front of you on the table. Place your hands palms down, your wrists at the edge of the table. Hold your elbows bent at 90 degrees. Line up your middle finger with the straight line of the L. Make sure an imaginary straight line runs through the mid-forearm and the middle finger. Then slide your wrist sideways toward the thumb side, keeping your forearm immobile. Do not (a) bend or extend your wrist up or down or (b) move your forearm (only the wrist). Now imagine a line running between the knuckle at the base of your middle finger and the middle of your wrist as it moves away from the line on the table. Repeat with the other wrist.

Record the following information for both wrists:

If this line moves past the midline between the two arms
    of the H shape, mark N.   _____
If it moves halfway or a little less, mark T.   _____
If it barely moves, mark TT.   _____

Compare sides:

If it hurt on both side, mark L/R.   _____
If it hurts more on one side, mark L or R.   _____
If there is no pain, mark N.   _____

Interpreting Your Results

If the range is *T* or *TT:* first, test the opposing muscles for tightness, the flexor carpi ulnaris and the extensor carpi ulnaris, which move the hand toward the little finger side (slow stretch).

Next, test the primary movers, the flexor carpi radialis (impaired function test) and the extensor carpi radialis, which move the hand toward the thumb side (impaired function test).

If the range is *N* but your muscles still ache, turn to Chapter 5, "Starting the Healing Process."

Standard Range: The wrist is able to move 25 degrees toward the thumb side.

Home Test 5: Bending the Fingers (Flexion)
Primary Mover: Flexor digitorum (brevis and longus)
Opposing Muscle: Extensor digitorum

Support your elbows on a table. Bend your arms at the elbow, keeping your wrists straight, with the fingers pointing to the ceiling. Turn your palms so they face each other. Make sure your hands and forearms are not rotated. Do not (a) bend your hand at the wrist either forward or backward, or (b) rotate the forearm or wrist. Look at one hand at a time.

Base of the Fingers Joint (Brevis)
Bend the fingers from the base, keeping them straight.
Record the following information for both hands:

If they bend all the way to a right angle (90 degrees) from
   their base, mark N.   _____
If the line of your fingers only can move past the midline
   between straight up and 90 degrees, mark T.   _____
If your fingers only move to this midline or less, mark TT.   _____

Standard Range: The fingers are able to bend to 90 degrees.

Middle joint (Longus)
Each finger may be different, so it is best to test each one separately. Start from the same position. Now curl your finger only at the middle joint, keeping the base joint straight.
Record the following information for each finger:

If the joint bends to more than a right angle (90 degrees),
   mark N.   _____

If the joint bends to a right angle (90 degrees), mark T. _____

If your finger bends less than a right angle, mark TT. _____

Standard Range: The middle joint can bend to 120 degrees.

Outer Joint

Start in the same position as above. Bend the middle joint to 90 degrees, then bend the outer joint.

Record the following information for each finger:

If the outer joint bends almost to a right angle, mark N. _____

If it bends to half of a right angle (45 degrees), mark T. _____

If it barely bends, mark TT. _____

Standard Range: 80 degrees for all.

Compare fingers and hands:

If it hurts on both sides, mark L/R. _____

If it hurts more or only on one side, one finger, or one
   hand, mark L/R and note which finger or hand.

If there is no pain, mark N. _____

Interpreting Your Results

If the range is *T* or *TT*: first, test the opposing muscles for tightness: the extensor digitorum, which straightens the fingers (slow stretch).

Next, test the primary mover, the flexor digitorum, which bends the fingers (impaired function test).

If the range is *N* but your muscles still ache, turn to Chapter 5, "Starting the Healing Process."

Home Test 6: Lifting the Fingers (Extension)

Primary Mover: Extensor digitorum

Opposing Muscle: Flexor digitorum

Support your elbows on a table close together, and press your palms and forearms against each other. Bend your arms at the elbow with straight wrists and fingers pointing to the ceiling. Make sure the joints at the base of the fingers are held together also. Bend your fingers backward away from the centerline as far as they go, one hand at a time (hold the other side straight up). Do not (a) move the base of your fingers apart or (b) move your hands from a symmetrical position.

Record the following information for each hand:

If the fingers of one hand move one and a half inches away
from the centerline, mark N. _____

If they move a half inch, mark T. _____

If they barely move away from the centerline, mark TT. _____

Compare sides:

If it hurts on both sides, mark L/R. _____

If it hurts more on one side, mark L or R. _____

If any of the fingers hurt more than the others, mark which
fingers. _____

Interpreting Your Results

If the range is *T* or *TT:* first, test the opposing muscle for tightness, the flexor digitorum, which bends the fingers (slow stretch).

Next, test the primary mover, the extensor digitorum, which straightens the fingers (impaired function test).

If the range is *N* but your muscles still ache, turn to Chapter 5, "Starting the Healing Process."

Standard Range: The fingers can bend backward to 30 degrees.

Home Test 7: Extending the Thumb out to the Side (Extension)

Primary Movers: Extensor pollicis brevis and longus
Opposing Muscles: Flexor pollicis brevis and longus

Place your hands palms down on the table, with your wrists on the edge of the table and all fingers pointing straight ahead. Do not slide from this position during the test. Slowly move the thumb out to one side as far as it will go. Do not (a) bend your thumb, (b) move your wrist, or (c) let your hand slide sideways.

Record the following information for each thumb:

If your thumb and index finger make an L shape, mark N. _____

If your thumb makes a wide V shape with the index finger,
   mark T.   _____
If your thumb makes a narrow V shape with the index finger,
   mark TT.   _____

Compare sides:

If it hurts on both sides, mark L/R.   _____
If it hurts more on one side, mark L or R.   _____
If there is no discomfort, mark N.   _____

Interpreting Your Results

If the range is *T* or *TT:* first, test the opposing muscles for tightness, the adductor pollicis and opponens pollicis, which bring the thumb across the palm of the hand (slow stretch).

Next, test the primary movers, the extensor pollicis longus and brevis, which reach the thumb out to the side (impaired function test).

If the range is *N* but your muscles still ache, turn to Chapter 5, "Starting the Healing Process."

Standard Range: The inner knuckle of the thumb is able to make an L shape with the thumb and index finger (which is really only 70 degrees range of motion, measuring the movement of the first thumb knuckle).

Home Test 8: Moving the Thumb Inward across the Palm (Flexion and Adduction)

Primary Movers: Adductor pollicis and opponens pollicis
Opposing Muscles: Extensor pollicis brevis and longus

Place your hand palm up on a table. Reach your thumb out to the side. From there, move your straight thumb slowly back in and across the palm. Try to keep your thumb close to the palm the entire time. Do not bend your wrist or cup your hand. You should be able to reach the base of your little finger with no discomfort. Repeat with the other hand.

Record the following information for both thumbs:

If your thumb reaches all the way across to the base of your
   little finger, mark N.   _____
If your thumb stops at the base of the fourth finger, mark T.   _____
If your thumb stops midway across the hand, mark TT.   _____

Compare sides:

If it hurts on both sides, mark L/R.   _____

If it hurts more on one side, mark L or R.   _____

If there is no pain, mark N.   _____

Interpreting Your Results

If the range is *T* or *TT*: first, test the opposing muscles for tightness, the extensor pollicis longus and brevis, which reach the thumb out to the side (slow stretch).

Next, test the primary movers, the adductor pollicis and opponens pollicis, which bring the thumb in and across the palm (impaired function test).

If the range is *N* but your muscles still ache, turn to Chapter 5, "Starting the Healing Process."

Standard Range: 15 degrees (measures the motion of the knuckle at the base of the thumb).

Tests for the Trunk

It is best to test these easily tensed muscles very slowly and gently.

Home Test 1: Bending Forward (Flexion)

Primary Mover: Rectus abdominis
Opposing Muscle: Erector spinae

In the starting position, let your arms hang relaxed at your side. Now move your hands a little in front of you so that they rest palms down on the front of your thighs. Slowly, releasing vertebra by vertebra (relax while you do this), let your fingertips slide down your legs as you bend forward until the fingertips are as close to the floor as possible. Do not (a) hyperextend or bend the knees, or (b) place feet closer or farther than four to five inches apart.

Record the following information:

If your fingertips or palms touch the floor, mark N.   _____

If your fingertips stop anywhere near halfway between
   the knees and toes, mark T.   _____

If your fingertips stop at the bottom of your knee, mark TT.
   (A great many people are unable to reach their toes.)   _____

Compare sides:

If it hurts on both sides, mark L/R.   _____

If it hurts more on one side, mark L or R.   _____

If there is no pain, mark N.   _____

Interpreting Your Results

If the range is *TT* or *T:* first, test the opposing muscle for tightness, the erector spinae, which bends the torso backward (slow stretch).

Next, test the primary mover, the rectus abdominis, which bends the torso forward (impaired function test).

If the range is *N* but your muscles still ache, turn to Chapter 5, "Starting the Healing Process."

Note: Gravity helps the body to bend forward. Therefore, weakness does not limit this motion in this position. Many people have weak abdominal muscles.

Standard Range: The trunk is able to bend 80 degrees toward the floor. This range is measured *after* the hip joint has bent to 90 degrees. When you bend to pick up something from the floor, it feels as if you have a huge range of motion. However, most of this motion is not happening in the spine. The motion stems from the joint of the thighbone and the hipbone. This joint does more than 50 percent of the back's forward bending. The standard range is correct only if the hip movement is not restricted by the muscles that straighten the hip, the hamstrings. If these are tight, the whole range of the back is limited. Therefore, to get a correct range of motion measurement for the back, we need to make sure that tight hamstrings are not a factor.

Test for Tight Hamstrings: Lie on your back and put your legs up against a wall, feet pointing to the ceiling. You should be able to be in a perfect 90-degree angle formed by your legs and trunk and not feel discomfort or tightness in the back of the thighs. If you any tightness in your hamstrings you need to subtract this from the range of the back (see page 228 for testing hamstring range).

Home Test 2: Bending Backward (Extension)

Primary Mover: Erector spinae
Opposing Muscle: Rectus abdominis

Lie on the floor on your stomach with your arms outstretched overhead. Grasp each arm just above the elbow with the opposite hand. Slide your elbows toward your body until they are directly under the shoulders while your torso bends up and backward as far as it gets. Do not (a) lift your hips off the floor or (b) stay in an extended backward posture for very long.

Record the following information:

If your elbows go all the way to 90 degrees, mark N.   _____

If your elbows slide to only halfway between the starting
    point and 90 degrees, mark T.   _____

If your elbows barely move, mark TT.   _____

Compare sides:

If it hurts on both sides, mark L/R.   _____

If it hurts more on one side, mark L or R.   _____

If there is no pain, mark N.   _____

Interpreting Your Results

If the range is *TT* or *T:* first, test the opposing muscle, for tightness, the rectus abdominis, which bends the torso forward (slow stretch).

Next, test the primary mover, the erector spinae, which bends the torso backward (impaired function test).

If the range is *N* but your muscles still ache, turn to Chapter 5, "Starting the Healing Process."

Standard Range: The trunk is able to bend 30 degrees backward.

Home Test 3: Bending the Trunk Sideways (Lateral Flexion)
Primary Mover: Quadratus lumborum on the same side
Opposing Muscle: Quadratus lumborum on the opposite side

You will need a roll of Scotch tape for this. Stand in the starting position and let your arms hang by your sides. Notice where the tips of the fingers are on the thighs, and mark this spot with a piece of tape. Bend slowly sideways as far as you can go, slightly lifting the opposite arm (bent at the elbow). Do not rotate the trunk. Again, mark the spot where your fingertips stop with tape. Measure the distance between the pieces of tape, the difference between the starting and ending positions. Repeat for the other side.

Record the following information for both sides:

If there is a six-inch difference, mark N.   _____

If there is a four-inch difference, mark T.   _____

If there is a two-inch difference, mark TT.   _____

Compare sides:

> If it hurts on both sides, mark L/R.   ———
> If it hurts more on one side, mark L or R.   ———
> If there is no pain, mark N.   ———

Interpreting Your Results

If the range is *TT* or *T*: first, test the opposing muscle for tightness, the quadratus lumborum on the opposite side, which bends the torso to the same side and opposes bending to the opposite side (slow stretch).

Next, test the primary mover, the quadratus lumborum on the same side, which bends the torso to the same side (impaired function test).

If the range is *N* but your muscles still ache, turn to Chapter 5, "Starting the Healing Process."

Note: Gravity helps to tilt the body to the side, so weakness does not limit this motion much.

Standard Range: The average range is 30 degrees. Most people are able to reach the knee joint.

Home Test 4: Rotating the Trunk (Rotation)

Primary Movers: Latissimus dorsi, abdominal and deep back muscles on the same side

Opposing Muscles: Latissimus dorsi, abdominal and deep back muscles on the other side

You will need a pencil for this test. Sit backward on a chair, with one leg on each side of the seat while you face the back of the chair. To help you observe the range, hold a pencil in the indentation where the collarbones meet in front, pointing the pencil straight ahead over the center of the back of the chair. Turn your torso to one side. Keep your elbows at your sides and your shoulders steady. Do not (a) move your hips, shoulders, or arms or (b) bend your torso. Make a note of how far out to the side along the back of the chair the pencil points after you have turned your trunk as far as you can. Repeat with the other side.

Record the following information for both sides:

> If the pencil moves six to eight inches away from the center of the
>   back of the chair, mark N.   ———
> If the pencil moves three to four inches away, mark T.   ———
> If the pencil moves one to two inches away, mark TT.   ———

Compare sides:

    If it hurts on both sides, mark L/R.

    If it hurts more on one side, mark L or R.   _____

    If there is no pain, mark N.   _____

Interpreting Your Results

If the range is *TT* or *T:* first, test the opposing muscles for tightness, the latissimus dorsi, abdominal and deep back muscles on the other side, which rotate the torso to their side and oppose rotating to the opposite side (slow stretch).

    Next, test the primary movers, the latissimus dorsi and the abdominal and deep back muscles on the same side, which rotate the torso to the same side (impaired function test).

    If the range is *N* but your muscles still ache, turn to Chapter 5, "Starting the Healing Process."

Standard Range: The trunk is able to turn 40 to 45 degrees.

Tests for the Hips and the Thighs

Home Test 1: Bending the Hip (Flexion)

Primary Movers: Iliopsoas, rectus femoris (one of the quads)
Opposing Muscles: Gluteus maximus, hamstrings

Lie on your back on the floor with your legs straight out and your hands on the floor. Bend one leg, bringing the knee toward your chest. Bend the knee as far as it will go. Keep your buttocks and other leg on the floor. Do not (a) lift your buttocks off the floor, (b) bend the other knee, or (c) rotate your body. Repeat with the other leg.

    Record the following information for both sides:

    If your knee points halfway between straight up to the
       ceiling and touching your chest, mark N.

    If your knee points almost straight up to the ceiling, mark T. _____

    If your knee points straight to the ceiling, mark TT.   _____

Compare sides:

    If it hurts on both sides, mark L/R.

    If it hurts more on one side, mark L or R.   _____

    If there is no pain, mark N.   _____

Interpreting Your Results

If the range is *TT* or *T*: first, test the opposing muscles for tightness, the gluteus maximus and hamstrings, which straighten and bend the body backward at the hip (slow stretch).

Next, test the primary movers, the iliopsoas and rectus femoris, which bend the body forward at the hip (impaired function test).

If the range is *N* but your muscles still ache, turn to Chapter 5, "Starting the Healing Process."

Standard Range: The hip is able to bend 115 to 125 degrees with the knee bent.

Home Test 2: Straightening the Hip and Bending Backward (Extension)

Primary Movers: Gluteus maximus, hamstrings
Opposing Muscles: Iliopsoas, rectus femoris

This test requires considerable strength. You can also test this range standing. Lie on your stomach on the floor, making sure both hipbones remain on the floor. Keep your knees straight and lift one leg. Try to turn your head so you can watch the knee's elevation off the floor. Do not (a) bend your lower back or knee, or (b) tilt the hip forward. Repeat with the other leg.

Record the following information for both sides:

If your leg lifts eight to ten inches off the floor, mark N.   _____
If your leg lifts only a few inches off the floor, mark T.   _____
If you cannot lift the leg at all, mark TT.   _____

Compare sides:

If it hurts on both sides, mark L/R.   _____
If it hurts more on one side, mark L or R.   _____
If there is no pain, mark N.   _____

To test the range standing, stand in the starting position. Place your hands on your hips to make sure the hip bowl does not move, only the thighbone, as you slowly move the toes (straight leg) backward until the foot stops. Keep your tailbone tucked in as you do this. Use the same measurements as above: eight inches, a few inches, and almost none.

Interpreting Your Results

If the range is *TT* or *T:* first, test the opposing muscles for tightness, the iliopsoas and the rectus femoris, which bend the body forward at the hip (slow stretch).

Next, test the primary movers, the gluteus maximus and the hamstrings, which straighten and bend the body backward at the hip (impaired function test).

If the range is *N* but your muscles still ache, turn to Chapter 5, "Starting the Healing Process."

Standard Range: The hip is able to move 30 degrees backward.

Home Test 3: Rotating the Leg Outward (External Rotation)

Primary Movers: Piriformis, gluteus maximus (of the key muscles)
Opposing Muscles: Gluteus minimus (not a key muscle), gluteus medius—front part, tensor fasciae latae

You will need Scotch tape for this test. Lie on your back on the floor with the soles of your feet flat against a wall. Place your hands on the hipbones so you can feel them moving, and be sure to keep your legs and knees straight and your foot in line with your knee. Mark the starting position of your toes (straight up) with tape. Rotate the entire legs (not the ankles) outward, keeping your heels together. Mark with tape where your toes end. It is very important to keep your knees and feet straight and in line so that you measure the rotation of the hip and not the ankle. Do not (a) move or rotate your ankle instead of the leg, or (b) rotate the pelvis (keep both bones on the floor).

Record the following information for both sides:

If your foot moves halfway to the floor (45 degrees), mark N.   _____
If your foot moves down two inches from the top, mark T.   _____
If your foot moves down one inch, mark TT.   _____

Compare sides:

If it hurts on both sides, mark L/R.   _____
If it hurts more or only on one side, mark L or R.   _____
If there is no pain, mark N.   _____

You can also do this test while standing: With your feet six inches apart and your hands on your hips to make sure they are stable, rotate one foot outward, keeping the sole on the floor, as far as it will go without moving the rest of the body. Watch the angle formed by the foot as it moves from straight ahead to the side. The same degrees apply.

Interpreting Your Results

If the range is *TT* or *T*: first, test the opposing muscles for tightness, the gluteus medius and tensor fasciae latae, which rotate the hip and thigh inward (slow stretch).

Next, test the primary movers, the piriformis and the gluteus maximus, which rotate the hip and thigh outward (impaired function test).

If the range is *N* but your muscles still ache, turn to Chapter 5, "Starting the Healing Process."

Standard Range: The hip is able to rotate outward to an angle of 45 degrees.

Home Test 4: Rotating the Leg Inward (Internal Rotation)

Primary Movers: Gluteus minimus (not a key muscle) gluteus medius (front part), tensor fasciae latae

Opposing Muscles: Piriformis, gluteus maximus (of the key muscles)

You will need Scotch tape for this test. Lie on your back on the floor with your feet against the wall, heels a little apart. As in the previous test, mark your foot's starting point with tape. Keep your hands on your hips so you can feel them move while you rotate one knee and leg straight inward as far as it will go. Be sure to keep your foot in line with your knee, and mark the ending point with tape. Do not (a) rotate the pelvis, (b) bend the trunk, or (c) turn the hip inward by lifting it.

You can also do this standing, with your feet eight inches apart this time and your hands on your hips to make sure they do not move—only the thighbone should rotate. Turn a foot inward, keeping the sole on the floor. Remember to keep your leg straight. Note the difference, and repeat with the other leg.

Record the following information for both sides:

If this action moves your foot halfway to the floor
    (45 degrees), mark N.   _____
If your foot moves two inches, mark T.   _____
If your foot moves one inch, mark TT.   _____

Compare sides:

> If it hurts on both sides, mark L/R.   _____
> If it hurts more on one side, mark L or R.   _____
> If there is no pain, mark N.   _____

Interpreting Your Results

If the range is *TT* or *T:* first, test the opposing muscles for tightness, the piriformis and the gluteus maximus, which rotate the hip and thigh outward (slow stretch).

Next, test the primary movers, the gluteus medius and the tensor fasciae latae, which rotate the hip and thigh inward (impaired function test).

If the range is *N* but your muscles still ache, turn to Chapter 5, "Starting the Healing Process."

Standard Range: The hip is able to rotate 45 degrees inward.

Home Test 5: Moving the Legs Apart (Hip Abduction)

Primary Movers: Gluteus medius, tensor fasciae latae (of the key muscles)
Opposing Muscles: Adductor magnus brevis and longus

Lie on your back on the floor, making sure both buttocks are on the floor and both legs point straight down along a midline. Move one leg out to the side, away from the midline, as far as it goes. Do not (a) rotate your hip outward, (b) tilt the hip, or (c) move the other leg. Repeat with the other leg.

Record the following information for both sides:

> If your leg goes out further than half of a right angle
>   (more than 45 degrees), mark N.   _____
> If your leg goes out half of a right angle (45 degrees),
>   mark T.   _____
> If your leg goes one-third of a right angle (30 degrees),
>   mark TT.   _____

Compare sides:

> If it hurts on both sides, mark L/R.   _____
> If it hurts more on one side, mark L or R.   _____
> If there is no pain, mark N.   _____

Interpreting Your Results

If the range is *TT* or *T*: first, test the opposing muscles for tightness, the adductors, which move the thighs in toward the body (slow stretch).

Next, test the primary movers, the gluteus medius and the tensor fasciae latae, which move the thigh out to the side (impaired function test).

If the range is *N* but your muscles still ache, turn to Chapter 5, "Starting the Healing Process."

Standard Range: The hip is able to move out to the side at 45 to 55 degrees.

Home Test 6: Pulling the Legs Together (Adduction)

Primary Mover: Adductor magnus
Opposing Muscles: Gluteus medius, tensor fasciae latae

Lie on your back on the floor with legs and knees straight. Keep your hands on your hips so that you can feel if they lift off the floor. Lift one leg slightly and cross it over the other, keeping both legs straight and watching the midline as you move. Do not (a) let the hip of the moving leg rise off the floor, (b) bend your knees, or (c) rotate the hip in. Repeat with the other leg.

Record the following information for both legs:

If your foot moves over easily and there is distance
    between your feet, mark N.   _____
If your foot moves across but the heels end up right
    next to each other, mark T.   _____
If you cannot move the foot across, mark TT.   _____

Compare sides:

If it hurts on both sides, mark L/R.   _____
If it hurts more on one side, mark L or R.   _____
If there is no pain, mark N.   _____

Interpreting Your Results

If the range is *TT* or *T*: first, test the opposing muscles for tightness, the gluteus medius and the tensor fasciae latae, which move the thigh out to the side (slow stretch).

Next, test the primary mover, the adductor magnus, which moves the thigh in toward the middle (impaired function test).

If the range is *N* but your muscles still ache, turn to Chapter 5, "Starting the Healing Process."

Standard Range: The hip is able to move in from the midline at an angle of 30 degrees.

Home Test 7: Sideways Tilt (Pelvic Imbalance)

You will need a pen and a ruler for this test. Stand in front of a mirror and look for your hipbones. If you cannot see them, feel with your hands until you find the bones in front. Mark the bones with a pen, making sure you mark both in exactly the same place. Use a stick or a ruler to see if the line between the two marks is level. Note if it is straight, or tilted to the right or left.

Interpreting Your Results

If there is a tilt, look for the muscles that hike the hip, the quadratus lumborum. Are they tight on the side of the higher hip? Can you bend to full range on both sides?

Home Test 8: Forward Tilt (Anterior Pelvic Tilt)

You will need a front mirror and a side mirror so you can see your profile. Refer to the drawing of aligned posture and correct back curve on page 37. Standing in the starting position, observe your lower back curve. Is it too deep? Most often, people have an anterior tilt due to weak abdominal muscles and excess abdominal weight.

Interpreting Your Results

If your lower back curve is too deep, look at the muscles that might be causing an anterior tilt. These are the rectus abdominus, which might be weak, and the rectus femoris, the erector spinae, the latissimus dorsi, and the quadratus lumborum, which might be tight. Stretches will help lengthen muscles and let the hip fall back to the aligned position.

Home Test 9: Backward Tilt (Posterior Pelvic Tilt)

Refer to the drawing of aligned posture showing the optimal back curve. Standing in the starting position, observe the curve of the lower back. Is it too flat? You can also lie on the floor: is there a space between your lower back and the floor?

Interpreting Your Results

Look at the muscles that bend the trunk and the hip forward, the iliopsoas, the quadratus lumborum, and the hamstrings. If tight, these can tilt the hip bowl backward.

Home Test 10: One Forward/One Backward Tilt (Anterior/Posterior Pelvic Tilt)

Standing in front of a mirror, find the two hipbones. Is one more prominent than the other? If so, the prominent side of the pelvis is pulled forward or the other side is pulled backward.

Interpreting Your Results

Are the hamstrings unevenly tight? (Do a stretch test.) Or is the iliopsoas tighter on one side than the other? (Do a stretch test.) If so, your hip bowl may be pulled forward on one side and back on the other. If the hamstrings are tight, the hip on that side is pulled backward, and if the iliopsoas is tight, the hip on that side is pulled forward.

Knee Tests

Home Test 1: Bending the Knee (Flexion)
Primary Movers: Hamstrings
Opposing Muscles: Quadriceps

Lie face down on the floor. Bend your knees to a right angle. (Turn your head and verify.) Next, bend one knee by bringing the heel toward your buttocks. Do not start without placing the knees in a right-angle position. Repeat with the other knee.

Record the following information for both heels:

If your heel goes halfway to your buttocks or more, mark N.   _____

If your heel moves halfway or less, mark T.   _____

If your heel barely moves, mark TT.   _____

Compare sides:

If it hurts on both sides, mark L/R.   _____

If it hurts more on one side, mark L or R.   _____

If there is no pain, mark N.   _____

Interpreting Your Results

If the range is *TT* or *T:* first, test the opposing muscles for tightness, the quadriceps, which straighten the knee (slow stretch).

Next, test the primary movers, the hamstrings, which bend the knee (impaired function test).

If the range is *N* but your muscles still ache, turn to Chapter 5, "Starting the Healing Process."

Note: The strain on the hamstrings depends on whether the hip is bent or straight. Since these muscles extend over and work two joints, the hip and the knee, there is less strain on the muscles if the hip is straight. Lying on the floor takes away the hip work and allows us to isolate the knee work of the hamstrings to bending the knee only.

Standard Range: The knee is able to bend 130 to 150 degrees (90 + 40 to 60). *Note:* If you pull the leg toward your buttocks with your hands, it may go all the way. The joint allows this. But if you pull, you are not testing the muscles that operate the joint.

Home Test 2: Straightening the Knee (Extension)
Primary Movers: Quadriceps
Opposing Muscles: Hamstrings

2a. This test depends on the strength of your quads. Sit on a kitchen table or a counter with your feet dangling. Straighten your knee by tightening your thigh muscles. Do not (a) move anything other than your knee or (b) deviate from the straight line. Repeat with the other leg.

2b. Do this if your quads are too painful to do 2a. This actually also tests the opposite side for tightness. Lie on the floor along a straight line on the side of the leg you are testing. Align the hip and ankle with this line. Keep your knee a little bent. Now straighten your knee by tightening the muscles in front of the thigh.

Record the following information for both legs:

If your leg is straight, mark N.   _____
If your knee is a little bent, mark T.   _____
If your knee is visibly bent, mark TT.   _____

Compare sides:

If it hurts on both sides, mark L/R.   _____

If it hurts more on one side, mark L or R.   _____
If there is no pain, mark N.   _____

Interpreting Your Results

If the range is *TT* or *T:* first, test the opposing muscles for tightness, the hamstrings, which bend the knee (slow stretch).

Next, test the primary movers, the quadriceps, which straighten the knee (impaired function test).

If the range is *N* but your muscles still ache, turn to Chapter 5, "Starting the Healing Process."

Standard Range: The knee should straigten to 180 degrees.

Ankle Tests

Home Test 1: Bending the Foot Down–Pointing the Toes (Pointing, Plantar Flexion)

Primary Movers: Gastrocnemius, soleus (calf muscles)
Opposing Muscle: Tibialis anterior

Kneel on a carpet or a pad on the floor so that your knee is at a right angle to your body. Check the position of both ankles in back of you to make sure they are not rolled in or out.

Record the following information for both ankles:

If the front of the ankle is flat on the floor, mark N.   _____
If you have to push on the ankle to make it go down, mark T. _____
If only the toe touches the floor and the rest of the ankle is
   in the air, mark TT.   _____

Compare sides:

If it hurts on both sides, mark L/R.   _____
If it hurts more on one side, mark L or R.   _____
If there is no pain, mark N.   _____

Interpreting Your Results

If the range is *TT* or *T:* first, test the opposing muscles for tightness, the tibialis anterior, which lifts the foot up (slow stretch).

Next, test the primary movers, the gastrocnemius and the soleus (calf muscles), which bend the foot down (impaired function test).

If the range is *N* but your muscles still ache, turn to Chapter 5, "Starting the Healing Process."

Standard Range: The ankle can straighten to 45 degrees (when you point your foot).

Home Test 2: Bending the Foot up—Toes toward Your Shin (Dorsiflexion)
Primary Mover: Tibialis anterior
Opposing Muscles: Gastrocnemius, soleus (calf muscles)

This also depends on the strength of the primary mover. Sit on a chair so that you can create a right angle with your knees bent and your foot on the floor. Lift your foot while keeping the heel on the ground. Watch the ball of the foot. Do not (a) bend your toes, (b) rotate the foot, or (c) start in a position where the angle of the ankle is not 90 degrees. Repeat with the other foot.

Record the following information for both feet:

If your foot lifts two inches or more off the floor, mark N.   _____
If your foot lifts one inch off the floor, mark T.   _____
If you cannot lift your foot off the floor, mark TT.   _____

Compare sides:

If it hurts on both sides, mark L/R.   _____
If it hurts more on one side, mark L or R.   _____
If there is no pain, mark N.   _____

Interpreting Your Results

If the range is *TT* or *T:* first, test the opposing muscles for tightness, the gastrocnemius and the soleus (calf muscles), which bend the foot down (slow stretch).

Next, test the primary mover, the tibialis anterior, which lifts the foot up (impaired function test).

If the range is *N* but your muscles still ache, turn to Chapter 5, "Starting the Healing Process."

Standard Range: The foot can lift up 20 degrees.

CHAPTER 12

Stretching Your Key Muscles

There is a difference between the stretching descriptions you will find in this chapter and those you are used to getting. These are designed to let you experience and understand the principles behind stretching, which will help you to better understand and remember the stretches you have been given. You'll learn to become aware of your simple everyday movement patterns while you stretch. Once you understand them, you won't need to carry the descriptions around with you; rather, you can integrate them into your daily routine, where they will soon become second-nature, easy-to-use tools for relieving your stress.

How can you tell if you are doing it right? Any time you are in doubt, you can turn to Chapter 9 and look up the muscle you want to stretch, its job, and its attachments to the bones. This will tell you how to stretch (by moving the two tendon attachments further apart) and where to feel the stretch (right in the area between the two bone attachments). This is all you need to know. The purpose of thinking while you stretch is to increase the control of your body and the effect of the stretch. In this chapter the heading will tell you the job of the muscle you will be stretching.

Remember: muscles work in pairs of opposites. When one muscle contracts, the opposing muscle (the muscle that does the exact opposite) always gets stretched.

Always assume your starting position before stretching.

The Neck

Bending Forward (Flexion)
Primary Mover: Sternocleidomastoid
Opposing Muscles: Splenius capitis, splenius cervicis

The sternocleidomastoid's job is to bend the head forward when both muscles are working together. To stretch it, therefore, you must bend the head backward.

Because the sternocleidomastoid muscle also turns (rotates) the head to the side (when only one muscle is working), an additional stretch is to rotate the head to the side, as in looking over your shoulder. Do both sides.

To Make the Stretch Passive: With your fingertips, push your chin up as far as it will go, slowly and gently releasing your head and neck, vertebra by vertebra. Hold briefly and release back into the starting position. (The neck is not used to this position, so do not hold it for more than one deep breath.)

Next, stretch the part of the muscle that rotates the head. Cup your hand over one side of your chin and slowly push your head to the side as far as it will go. Repeat three or four times or until it feels as if the muscle has adapted.

Bending Backward (Extension)

Primary Movers: Splenius capitis, splenius cervicis
Opposing Muscle: Sternocleidomastoid

The job of the splenius muscles is to bend the head backward. To stretch them, therefore, you must bend your head forward.

To Make the Stretch Passive: From the starting position, tuck your chin in, lace your fingers behind your head, and push your head toward your chest. Let your head release first, then your neck, vertebra by vertebra, until you have reached your full range of motion. Hold for a couple of deep breaths and release back into the starting position. Repeat three or four times or until it feels as if the muscle has adapted.

Bending Sideways (Lateral Flexion)

Primary Movers: Scalenes
Opposing Muscles: Scalenes on the opposite side

The job of the scalenes is to bend the head toward your shoulder. To stretch them, therefore, you must bend the head to the other side. The scalenes also help to bend the head forward, so to stretch them fully you must also bend the head a little backward while bending it to the side.

To Make the Stretch Passive: In the starting position, place one hand over the top of your head, reaching over the ear on the other side. Then, slowly and gently, pull your head sideways so that your ear is drawn toward the shoulder. Hold and release back into the starting position. Repeat three or four times or until it feels as if the muscle has adapted.

The Shoulder

Shrugging and Depressing the Shoulder (the Trapezius)
Primary Mover: Upper trapezius
Opposing Muscle: Lower trapezius

The main job of the upper trapezius is to lift the shoulders. Therefore, to stretch it you must depress your shoulders. The upper trapezius also helps to bend the head and neck backward, so to stretch it fully you must bend the neck forward.

To Make the Stretch Passive: Sitting in the starting position, place your hand over your head and on the back of your skull and grab the seat of your chair behind your hip with the other hand. Now pull the back of your head forward and diagonally away from the shoulder of the arm that holds the chair. Feel the stretch between the tip of your shoulder and the back of your head. Hold for a couple of deep breaths and release. Repeat three or four times or until it feels as if the muscle has adapted.

Pulling the Shoulder Blade in toward the Spine
Primary Mover: Middle trapezius
Opposing Muscle: Pectoralis major

The main job of the middle trapezius is to pull the shoulder blade in toward the spine. Therefore, to stretch it you must pull your arm out and forward.

To Make the Stretch Passive: Stand in a doorway and hold onto each side of the doorway at shoulder height with straight arms. Slowly lean back as far as you can, keeping your hips straight. Feel the stretch between your upper spine and shoulder. Hold for a couple of deep breaths and release. Repeat three or four times or until it feels as if the muscle has adapted.

Depressing the Shoulder
Primary Mover: Lower trapezius
Opposing Muscle: Upper trapezius

The main job of the lower trapezius is to depress the shoulder. Therefore, to stretch this part, you must elevate the shoulder.

To Make the Stretch Passive: You can elevate your shoulders without using other muscles if you stand with your back against a counter or a stable table. Place both palms on the edge with your fingers hanging down. Keeping your hips straight, bend your knees, allowing your shoulders to be raised. Feel the stretch between the top of your shoulder blade and the middle spine. Repeat until you no longer feel a stretch.

Shrugging the Shoulders (Shoulder Elevation)

Primary Mover: Levator scapulae
Opposing Muscles: Lower trapezius, latissimus dorsi

The levator scapulae's job is to lift the shoulder. Therefore, to stretch it you must depress the shoulder. It also bends the neck to the side and backward, so to stretch it fully you must bend your neck to the other side and forward.

To Make the Stretch Passive: Sit on a chair in the starting position. Grab the seat of the chair behind your hip on the same side as the muscle being stretched. With your other hand, pull your head forward and away from the shoulder blade of the arm that is holding the chair. You can get a good grip if you bring your hand over your head and hold it over the ear. Feel the stretch between the shoulder blade and the side of the neck. To get this important stretch right, look up the location of the two attachment sites of the levator scapulae.

Pulling the Shoulders Back (Scapular Adduction)

Primary Movers: Rhomboids
Opposing Muscle: Pectoralis major

The rhomboids' job is to pull the shoulder blades toward the spine and ribs. Therefore, to stretch them you must pull the shoulder blades away from the spine (round your shoulders).

To Make the Stretch Passive: Sit on a chair in the starting position and lean your upper back and head forward, keeping your lower back and hips straight. Let your arms hang between your knees. If you fill your lungs with air and round your upper back up like a cat, you will feel the pull between the spine and the inner border of your shoulder blade (the two tendon sites).

Moving the Shoulder Blades away from the Spine (Scapular Abduction)

Primary Mover: Serratus anterior

Opposing Muscles: Rhomboids

The serratus anterior's job is to bring the shoulder blades away from the spine, which happens when the shoulders and arms are brought forward and up. Therefore, to stretch it you must raise your arm up behind your body and push so the shoulder blades are moved closer together.

To Make the Stretch Passive: Stand with your back to a counter. Place your palms on the edge of the counter, about a shoulder width apart, with your fingers over the edge. Keeping your hips straight, bend your knees to lower your body, and try to avoid bending forward. Lower yourself as far as you can, and feel the stretch under the shoulder blades and along the side of your trunk (the two tendon sites).

Raising the Arms (Flexion, Abduction, and Extension of the Shoulder)

Raising the Arm in Front
Primary Mover: Front part of the deltoid
Opposing Muscle: Back part of the deltoid

The job of the front part of the deltoid is to lift the arm up in front of the body. Therefore, to stretch it you must lift your arm up behind the body.

Raising the Arm up to the Side
Primary Mover: Middle part of the deltoid
Opposing Muscles: Pectoralis major, latissimus dorsi

The job of the middle part of the deltoid is to raise the arm out to the side. Therefore, to stretch it you must bring your arm down and in toward the body.

To Make the Stretch Passive (Front and Middle Part):   Bring both arms behind your back. Take hold of the back of one elbow and pull it gently farther across your back. Feel the stretch between the tip of the shoulder and the outside of the upper arm bone. Hold for a couple of deep breaths and release. Repeat until you feel the muscle has adapted. Shift sides.

Raising the Arm in Back
Primary Mover: Back part of the deltoid
Opposing Muscle: Front part of the deltoid, pectoralis major

The job of the back part of the deltoid is to lift the arm up behind the body. Therefore, to stretch it fully you must lift your arm up in front of the body.

To Make the Stretch Passive (Back Part):   Lift the arm up in front of your body with your elbow bent and pointing forward. With your other hand, reach under your upper arm, take hold of it, and pull it across your chest. Feel the pull between the back of the tip of your shoulder and the outside of the upper arm bone. Hold for a couple of deep breaths and release. Repeat until you feel the muscle has adapted. Shift sides.

Rolled-In Shoulders (Flexion, Adduction, and Internal Rotation of the Arm)
Primary Mover: Pectoralis major
Opposing Muscles: Rhomboids

The pectoralis major's job is to pull the arms in to the side and across your chest. Therefore, to stretch it you must pull your arms out to the side and back.

To Make the Stretch Passive: Stand in a doorway in a hands-up position. Place your elbows on both sides of the doorway, shoulder high, and push your arms and shoulders out to the side by leaning your torso forward in the doorway. It helps to place one foot in front of you and one behind you for balance. Feel the pull between the collarbone, upper arm bone, and chest (breastbone), where this muscle's tendons attach. Hold for a couple of deep breaths and release. You can also stretch one arm at a time: Assume the same position as above, with only one elbow on the doorframe. Twist your body away from this side. Doing one at the time gives you even more of a stretch.

Note: You can vary this doorway stretch so as to stretch every part of the front of your chest and shoulders by moving your arms a couple of inches up on the frame at a time, each time leaning your body through the doorway and doing a full stretch. When your arms are straight up you can move back down a little at the time, this time stretching with straight arms.

Working with the Arms behind the Back
Primary Mover: Latissimus dorsi
Opposing Muscles: Pectoralis major's upper part, upper trapezius

The latissimus dorsi's job is to lift the arm backward and up behind the body from a fully lifted position in front of the body. Therefore, to stretch it you must lift your arm forward and up. It also pulls the shoulder down, so to stretch it fully you must lift your shoulder blades.

To Make the Stretch Passive: Hang from a bar or grab onto a doorframe above your head and let your body hang. You should feel the stretch on the back of the upper arm and the side of the trunk as the stretch pulls the tendon sites farther apart. Another way to feel this stretch is to kneel in front of a chair an arm's length away with both hands on the seat. Keep your arms and back straight and your hips at 90 degrees. Push down on the seat and feel the stretch on the sides of your trunk and along the outside of your upper arm. Hold for a couple of deep breaths and release.

The Elbow

Bending the Elbow (Flexion)
Primary Mover: Brachioradialis
Note: The biceps is the primary mover for bending the arm at the elbow, but it is not a key muscle in this book.
Opposing Muscle: Triceps

The job of the brachioradialis is to bend the arm at the elbow and also to bring the forearm back to a neutral position between inward and outward rotation. Therefore, to stretch it you must straighten your arm and rotate your forearm inward. You can extend your arms straight out to the side and bend your wrist so your fingers point toward the floor. In this position, rotate your forearms and hands inward and around as far as they go so the fingers point toward the back. This is also a great stretch for all the hand and finger muscles in the forearm.

To Make the Stretch Passive: Let your arm hang down by your side, with the palm rotated inward and out to the side as far as you can. Hold onto the forearm right below the elbow and twist the forearm even more inward. Hold for a couple of deep breaths and release. Repeat until you feel the muscle has adapted.

Straightening the Elbow (Extension)
Primary Mover: Triceps
Opposing Muscle: Brachioradialis

The job of the triceps is to straighten the elbow. Therefore, to stretch it you must bend your elbow. The triceps also helps lift (extend) the arm backward, so to stretch it fully you must lift (flex) the arm up and forward.

To Make the Stretch Passive: With your elbow bent maximally and your arm raised toward the ceiling (the elbow is pointing to the ceiling), extend the other hand over your head. Hold onto the elbow and pull it straight backward. Feel the stretch between the elbow, the upper arm, and the shoulder blade. Hold for a couple of deep breaths and release.

Turning the Forearm Palm Down (Pronation)

Primary Mover: Pronator teres
Opposing Muscle: Supinator

The job of the pronator teres is to turn the forearm inward, palms down when elbows are kept at 90 degrees. To stretch it, therefore, you must rotate your forearm outward, palms up.

To Make the Stretch Passive: Bend the arm at the elbow with your fingers pointing toward the ceiling and with the palm facing the body. Grab the forearm right below your wrist and twist it outward toward the thumb side.

Turning the Forearm Palm Up (Supination)

Primary Mover: Supinator
Opposing Muscle: Pronator teres

The job of the supinator is to rotate the forearm outward, turning the hand palm up when your elbows are bent to 90 degrees. To stretch it, therefore, you must turn your forearm inward as far as it will go. The same stretch you did for the brachioradialis also works for the supinator. Hold your arms straight out to the side. In this position bend your wrist so your fingers point toward the floor. Slowly rotate your fingers until they point toward the back.

To Make the Stretch Passive: Letting your arm hang down by your side, with your other hand grab your forearm directly below your elbow and twist the forearm inward.

The Hand and Wrist

Bending the Hand (Flexion)

Primary Movers: Flexor carpi radialis and flexor carpi ulnaris

Opposing Muscles: Extensor carpi radialis and extensor carpi ulnaris

The job of the flexor carpi radialis is to bend the hand at the wrist. Therefore, to stretch it you must lift the hand at your wrist and bend it backward. The muscle also bends the wrist sideways toward the thumb side. Therefore, to stretch it fully you must bend the wrist sideways toward the little finger side.

To Make the Stretch Passive: Interlace your fingers as in prayer, turn the palms out, and straighten your arms fully. You can also stand by a table and place your hand palm down on the table, palm turned so your fingers point toward your body. With a straight arm gently put weight on the hand and lean away from the table (don't turn your body). Stretch one wrist at the time. Feel the stretch on the inside of your forearm where the muscles run up to the elbow. You can vary this stretch in many ways, as any bending of the hand away from the inside of your forearm will stretch these muscles.

To stretch the part of the muscle that bends the wrist sideways. While sitting, lean your elbow and forearm on your thigh with the palms facing up and your wrists hanging over your knee. Place your other hand palm down over the thumb on this hand and gently move your wrist sideways toward the little finger side. If at the same time you bend your wrist a little, you get a full stretch. *Note:* Your wrist is not used to this motion, so do not push hard. Experiment to get the hang of this subtle stretch.

Lifting the Hand (Extension)
Primary Movers: Extensor carpi ulnaris and extensor carpi radialis
Opposing Muscles: Flexor carpi ulnaris and flexor carpi ulnaris

The job of the extensor carpi ulnaris is to lift (extend) the hand at the wrist and help pull the hand sideways toward the little finger. Therefore, to stretch it you must bend (flex) the hand at the wrist and also pull the hand sideways toward the thumb.

To Make the Stretch Passive: While holding your arm straight out in front of you, bend your wrist so the fingers point toward the floor. With your other hand, grasp the hand of your outstretched arm and pull it toward your body. Depending on where you have tightness, you may feel the stretch along the back of your hand where the tendon passes, or along the outer side of the forearm up to where the elbow attaches. Another effective way to do this stretch is to stand by a table with your arm hanging down at your side, palm turned inward. Rotate the hands so the palms are facing away from the body. Bend your hand at the wrist with your fingers pointing straight to the side. This is the first half of the stretch. To increase the stretch, place the back of your hand on the table (don't turn your body) and with a straight arm, gently put weight on the hand. This can be a very strong stretch if you push too hard. You can also, while seated, sit on the tips of your fingers, palms turned in, and push your wrists toward the floor while you push your elbows forward.

As you see, there are many different ways to perform a stretch, yet they all move the two muscle attachments farther apart.

Tensing the Palm
Primary Mover: Palmaris longus
Opposing Muscles: Extensor carpi radialis, extensor carpi ulnaris, and extensor digitorum

The job of the palmaris longus is to bend the wrist and curl the fingers, making the hand into a claw. Therefore, to stretch it you must bend (extend) your wrist and hand away from the inside of your forearm and spread your fingers to stretch the inside of the palm.

To Make the Stretch Passive: Stand in front of a table with your arm by your side. Turn the palm so it faces forward. Spread your fingers wide and place your hand on the table with the fingers pointing away from the table. Gently put weight on the hand and lean your body away from your wrist. You can also spread your fingers and put your hands together, fingertip to fingertip, in front of you, keeping your elbows bent. Turn your hands so the fingertips point toward your body and push your palms together and away from the body.

Bending the Fingers (Flexion)
Primary Mover: Flexor digitorum
Opposing Muscle: Extensor digitorum

The job of these muscles is to bend the fingers (curl them) and to help bend (flex) the wrist. Therefore, to stretch them you must straighten the fingers and bend (extend) the wrist.

To Make the Stretch Passive: (1) Hold your arm straight out in front of you, with your forearm rotated outward, palms up. With the other hand, push the fingers down as far as they will go while you straighten the elbow to its limit. (2) Lean your elbow on a table while sitting. Bend your arm, point fingers toward the ceiling, and rotate your forearms so your palms face your body. To stretch the base joint of each finger, curl the finger you are going to stretch (this is so you can get a good grip with the other hand to push the finger away from the palm). With the other hand, hold the curled finger and firmly push it backward away from the palm. Do one finger at a time. Do the thumb straight. (3) Stand by a table, arms by your sides, and turn your palm so it faces the table. Place the palm of the hand on the table with the base of the fingers on the table edge. Straighten your elbow completely, and with the other hand lift each straight finger off the table.

Lifting the Fingers (Extension)

Primary Mover: Extensor digitorum
Opposing Muscle: Flexor digitorum

The extensor digitorum's job is to lift the fingers and also to help lift the hand at the wrist. Therefore, to stretch it fully you must bend both the fingers and the wrist.

To Make the Stretch Passive: (1) Let your arm hang straight down or raise it straight out in front of you. Bend (flex) your hand at the wrist. Place the other hand on the back of this hand and push the base of the fingers (the first row of knuckles) toward you, keeping your elbow straight. The fingers can alternately point down or in toward the middle. (2) Lean your elbow on a table, fingers pointing to the ceiling, palm facing away from the body. Bend (flex) your wrist, and curl the fingers. One at a time, with your other hand, push the second finger joint (second from the tip) closer to your palm. The finger must be curled while you do this. Feel the stretch over the back of your hand and down the wrist and forearm. Repeat with each finger.

Reaching the Thumb up and out to the Side (Extension)

Primary Mover: Extensor pollicis longus
Opposing Muscle: Adductor pollicis

The job of this muscle is to reach the thumb out to the side. Therefore, to stretch it you must bring your thumb in across the palm.

To Make the Stretch Passive: Support your forearm on a table or on the armrest of a chair, palm down. Bend (flex) the wrist. Curl your thumb. With the other hand, push the first knuckle of your thumb in across the palm. Allow the wrist to move in the same direction. If you use your thumb a lot you should feel a strong stretch along your thumb, across the wrist, and up half of your forearm.

Moving the Thumb in across the Palm (Adduction)
Primary Movers: Adductor pollicis and opponens pollicis
Opposing Muscles: Extensor, abductor pollicis

The job of these muscles is to bend the thumb and bring it in across the palm. To stretch it, therefore, you must bring the thumb out to the side.

To Make the Stretch Passive: (1) Support your elbow on a table, fingers pointing to the ceiling, with your palm facing away from your body. Bend your wrist back toward your body, and with the other hand, pull your thumb down toward the forearm. (2) Stand in front of a table with your forearm turned outward, palm facing forward, away from your body. Place your palm on the table with your fingers hanging over the edge. With the other hand, reach in front of this arm and gently pull the thumb out and up from the table.

The Trunk

Bending Forward (Flexion)
Primary Mover: Rectus abdominis
Opposing Muscle: Erector spinae

The job of the rectus abdominis is to bend the trunk forward. Therefore, to stretch it you must bend your trunk backward.

To Make the Stretch Passive: (1) You will need a bed with a firm mattress and a pile of firm pillows. Sit with your buttocks right on the edge of the bed. Lean back on the pillows. You should feel the stretch along the whole front of your abdomen. (2) Stand in a doorway. With bent elbows, place your forearms on each side of the doorframe at shoulder height. Place one foot a little forward and the other foot a little back of the door for balance. With most of your weight on your back foot, slowly release your hips forward (lowering the body somewhat). Don't arch your back, just lengthen the front. Little by little, push your lower and upper trunk forward. Feel the strong stretch from ribs to the lower hipbone in front. You must relax both hips and shoulders fully to do this stretch. Change the position of your feet.

Bending Backward (Extension)

Primary Mover: Erector spinae
Opposing Muscles: Rectus abdominis and iliopsoas

The job of the erector spinae is to bend the trunk backward. Therefore, to stretch it you must bend your trunk forward.

To Make the Stretch Passive: (1) Sit on the edge of a chair. Slowly lean your upper body forward with your arms hanging down between your legs, and carefully allow your head to drop toward the floor. Let your back release vertebra by vertebra. (2) Stand in front of a post, the doorknob of a locked door, or anything that you can hold onto securely with both hands in front of you. Place your hands, one above the other, on the post at a little under hip level. Position your feet one and a half to two feet away from the post. Bend your knees a little and slowly lean backward. Push your buttocks out and feel the stretch all along your back. You can lean first to one side and then the other to feel the stretch more on the sides. By bending your knees more or less, you can feel the stretch higher or lower in the back. (3) From the standing position, bend forward with your back rounded, your knees bent, and your arms out to the sides as if you're embracing a huge balloon in front of you. Bend your knees further to get closer to the floor, and make your back as broad as you can.

Bending the Trunk Sideways (Lateral Flexion)

Primary Mover: Quadratus lumborum
Opposing Muscle: Quadratus lumborum on the other side

The job of the quadratus lumborum is to bend the trunk to the same side and to help bend it backward. Therefore, to stretch it you must bend your trunk to the opposite side and forward.

To Make the Stretch Passive: Gravity helps make this stretch passive. Stand with your feet about one foot apart for good balance. Placing one hand behind your neck, lean to the opposite side, letting the free arm side slide down your thigh. Feel the stretch all along your side between the hipbone and the lowest rib (the two tendon sites). To stretch the muscle fully, bend a little forward after you have bent as far as you can to the side.

The Hip

Bending the Hip (Flexion)
Primary Mover: Iliopsoas
Opposing Muscles: Gluteus maximus and hamstrings

The job of the iliopsoas is to bend the body at the hip. Therefore, to stretch it you must straighten your body and bend your legs and body backward at the hip.

To Make the Stretch Passive: (1) Stand with your back to a table about three or four feet away. Position a chair so you can hold onto the back for support. Raise your leg up behind your body and place your toes (sole facing the ceiling) on the table; your knee should be only slightly bent. Hold onto the back of the chair. Push down and let the knee you are standing on bend just a little bit. Also bend your body a little back from the hips. Feel the stretch between the front (top) of your thigh and deep in the abdomen (the spine). Hold for a couple of deep breaths and release. Do the other side. (2) While standing in the starting position, hold your hands on your hips to make sure you keep the weight over your hips. Move one foot back, letting it slide along the floor with the leg straight. Without shifting your weight to your toe, lean your upper body backward and feel the stretch deep in your abdomen. Do the other side.

Straightening the Hip (Extension)
Primary Movers: Gluteus maximus and hamstrings
Opposing Muscles: Iliopsoas and rectus femoris (one of the quads)

The job of these two muscles is to straighten the hip. Therefore, to stretch them you must bend (flex) your hip.

To Make the Stretch Passive: The gluteus maximus (see stretch for hamstrings, page 248) is stretched anytime you sit down or bend forward. To stretch it to its fullest range, lie on the floor, bend one knee at the time, and pull it toward your chest as far as it will go. Hold for a couple of deep breaths and release.

Rotating the Leg Outward (External Rotation)

Primary Mover: Piriformis
Opposing Muscles: Gluteus minimus (not a key muscle), gluteus medius—front part, tensor fasciae latae

The job of the piriformis is to rotate the hip and the thigh out to the side. Therefore, to stretch it you must rotate your hip and the thigh inward.

To Make the Stretch Passive: Lie on the floor with your knees bent. Place one foot over the knee of the other leg, and with your heel push this knee toward the other leg and down toward the floor. Let the thigh rotate fully inward. Try not to lift your hips off the floor.

Pulling the Legs Together (Adduction)

Primary Movers: Adductors
Opposing Muscle: Gluteus medius

The job of the adductors is to bring the thighs together and help bend the hip. Therefore, to stretch them you must bring the thigh out to the side.

To Make the Stretch Passive: (1) Stand with your legs comfortably far apart, hands on your hips. Move your upper body sideways toward the other leg (keep the upper body straight) and let this knee bend. Feel the stretch along the inside of the thigh you are leaning away from. (2) An easy stretch is to lie against a wall with your legs up along the wall. Let the legs move apart and feel the stretch on the inside of your thighs.

Moving the Thighs Apart (Abduction)

Primary Mover: Gluteus medius
Opposing Muscles: Adductors

The gluteus medius's job is to move the thigh out to the side and also to rotate the thigh inward (front part). Therefore, to stretch it you must bring your thigh in toward the middle and rotate it outward.

To Make the Stretch Passive: Stand with your hands on your hips, fingers forward so you can feel the movement of the hips. Turn one foot so that the leg is rotated outward (you are stretching this leg's hip). Cross the other leg over and place one foot to the side and one foot more forward than the other. Gently push the hip you are stretching sideways as far as it will go. Feel the stretch between the outside of the hipbone and the top of the thighbone.

The following muscle moves both the hip and the knee, but it is not the primary mover for either:

Muscle: Tensor fasciae latae
Opposing Muscle: Gluteus maximus

The job of the tensor fasciae latae is to bend (flex) the hip, move the thigh out to the side, and rotate the thigh inward. Therefore, to stretch it you must straighten your hip, move your thigh in, and rotate the thigh outward.

To Make the Stretch Passive: (1) Stand sideways by a counter or a table for support. Cross your outer leg over the other and place its foot on the floor. Allow the inner hip to tilt up a little. Next, slowly bend backward as you gently push this hip forward and a little toward the counter. You should feel the stretch in front of your hipbone, a little to the side, and down the top of the thigh. (2) Lie on your back on the edge of a bed, with the hip and the thigh you want to stretch just off the side of the bed. Roll this hip slightly outward away from the edge and you should feel the stretch on the front and side of the hipbone as well as down the upper thigh.

The Knee

Bending the Knee (Flexion)
Primary Movers: Hamstrings
Opposing Muscles: Quadriceps

The job of the hamstrings is to bend the knee and straighten the hip. Therefore, to stretch them you must straighten your knee and bend your body at the hip.

To Make the Stretch Passive: (1) You will need a belt, a rope, or a towel. Lie on your back on the floor. Bend one knee and put the rope around your foot. Slowly straighten your knee all the way, keeping your leg up in the air. If you can, continue pulling the foot and leg toward your body after the knee is straight. By turning your foot outward and inward while stretching, you will stretch the outer and inner parts of the hamstrings. (2) You will need a chair or low table and a towel. Kneel by the side of the chair or the table, with the towel under your knees and your hand on the seat or table for balance. Stretch one leg forward and move the other knee backward as far as comfortable. Lean on the forward leg and stretch as close to the splits position as you can. (3) The easy way—stand a foot away from a table or a desk that can resist your slight pulling. Bend forward with a straight back. Take hold of the edge of the surface and push your buttocks away from it. Feel the stretch between the hipbone inside your buttocks and the back of your knee, where the two tendon sites are. Hold for a couple of deep breaths and release. Repeat until you feel the muscle has adapted.

Straightening the Knee (Extension)
Primary Movers: Quadriceps
Opposing Muscles: Hamstrings

The job of the quadriceps is to straighten the knee and also to bend the hip (only one of the quads does this—the rectus femoris). Therefore, to stretch the quads you must bend your knees and straighten your hip.

To Make the Stretch Passive: Sit on your knees and put your hands on the floor behind you. Walk your hands slowly backward until you feel the strong stretch in your thighs. This stretches four of the quadriceps muscles. To fully stretch the two-joint muscle (rectus femoris) that bends the hip, stand up and lift your heel so you can grab around your ankle and pull the heel toward your buttocks. If you turn your foot outward and inward while stretching, you can stretch different parts of the quads, just as you did with the hamstrings.

Bending the Foot Down—Pointing the Toes (Plantar Flexion)
Primary Mover: Calf muscles
Opposing Muscle: Tibialis anterior

The job of the calf muscles is to bend the foot down, as in pointing the foot. Therefore, to stretch them you must bend your foot upward toward the shin of your leg.

To Make the Stretch Passive: Stand on a step on a stairway with your toes on the edge of the stair. Let your body weight slowly lower your heels down so the toes are brought closer to the shin of the lower leg. Straighten your knees fully and feel the stretch along the back of the lower leg.

Bending the Foot Up—Toes toward Your Shin (Dorsiflexion)

Primary Mover: Tibialis anterior
Opposing Muscle: Calf muscle

The job of the tibialis anterior is to bend the foot up. Therefore, to stretch it you must bend your foot down, pointing your foot.

To Make the Stretch Passive: Sit on your knees, leaning your body weight on your lower leg and ankle, so the top of the foot is flat against the floor.

Turning the Sole of the Foot out to the Side (Eversion)

Primary Mover: Peroneus longus and brevis
Opposing Muscle: Tibialis anterior

The job of the peroneus is to turn the sole of the foot out to the side, and also to help bend the foot down, as in pointing your foot. Therefore, to stretch it you must turn the sole of your foot inward, inverting it, and bend it up.

To Make the Stretch Passive: Sit on a chair. Moving one foot at the time, invert the foot while at the same time bending it up. You can also put your foot on the floor and, with the weight from your leg, carefully roll the outer side of the foot onto the floor, inverting it further.

Lifting the Toes (Extension)

Primary Movers: Extensor digitorum longus, extensor hallucis longus
Opposing Muscle: Flexor hallucis longus

The job of these muscles is to lift the toes and help bend the foot up. Therefore, to stretch them you must curl your toes and bend your foot down.

To Make the Stretch Passive: Sit on a chair or on the floor with your knees bent. Place the heel of the foot that you want to stretch on your other knee, and grab the toes with your hand. Pull the toes downward into a curl, and continue pulling the foot down until you feel the stretch up the front of your lower leg.

CHAPTER 13

Strengthening Your Key Muscles

The point of strengthening a muscle based on and focusing on the job it does is that you can do exactly what is necessary without involving a lot of unnecessary muscles. If you eliminate the unassigned helping muscles, the primary muscle works more effectively.

Many of the exercises may seem to require no effort at all. The purpose of this program is not to build muscle bulk, but to observe your muscles and to strengthen them so as to achieve pain-free, even, and balanced cooperation between the muscles in the body.

You should consider the weights and number of repetitions suggested as guidelines for a beginning program. If you have trouble managing the suggested amount, don't despair. Use this as a goal to work up to, and begin only with what you can do comfortably. Others may need to increase the weight or double the repetitions to really work the muscles.

The reason you should not go right to strengthening, but take a little time first to test your muscle, is that you can add to your problems quite effectively if you strengthen a muscle that is not ready. Therefore, if your muscles are tight and painful, stop the tests and the strengthening exercises as soon as you feel pain. Take time to heal before you proceed with strengthening.

Remember: Muscles work in pairs of opposites. When one muscle is strengthened, it always affects the balance between it and the other muscles in the group (the opposing and assisting muscles).

Start each test and exercise from your safe starting position.

The Neck

Bending Forward (Flexion)
Primary Mover: Sternocleidomastoid
Opposing Muscles: Splenius capitis and splenius cervicis

The sternocleidomastoid's job is to bend the head forward and rotate the head to the opposite side. Gravity aids this muscle in its job; likewise, to strengthen it you can make use of gravity to add resistance.

To Test: Lying on your back on the floor, lift your head, tucking your chin in. Lift as far as your pain-free range allows, and then lower your head back down to the floor. Repeat five times.

To Strengthen: Lying on your back on the floor, lift your head and neck toward your chest and then lower them down again (gravity provides the resistance). Lift and lower three times, lowering the head and neck very slowly the last time. To strengthen the muscle fully, do the same lying on your side and rotating your head to the opposite side. *Alternative:* Sit in a chair and position your hand on your forehead as you push your head forward against it, using your hand to resist the movement of your head. Similarly, place your hand on your cheek and push as you try to rotate your head toward it.

Bending Backward (Extension)
Primary Movers: Splenius capitis and splenius cervicis
Opposing Muscle: Sternocleidomastoid

The job of the splenius capitis and the splenius cervicis is to bend the head backward and to help bend the head to the same side.

To Test: *Splenius capitis* (lifts the head only): Lie on your stomach on a bed. Scoot forward so that your chin is just far enough over the edge of the bed that it allows your head and neck to bend. Feel the neck being stretched. Lift your head and neck up as high as your pain-free range allows. Look at the wall in front of you. Lower back down. Repeat five times.

To Strengthen: Lying on your stomach on the bed, in the same way lift and lower your head and neck three times, lowering them as slowly as you can the last time (gravity provides resistance). Repeat this sequence three times. *Alternative:* Sit in a chair and lace your hands behind your head. Push forward with your hands as you try to bend your head and neck backward.
   Splenius cervicis (lifts the neck from where it attaches on the spine, between the shoulder blades): Lie on your bed. Scoot forward so that your shoulders are about three inches off the edge. This allows your head to

hang down so you can look under the bed. Feel the stretch from between the shoulder blades and up the neck. As you lift, concentrate your mind on the spot on the neck between the shoulder blades and lift slowly up while you keep looking at the floor (do not look at the wall). Test and strengthen using the same sequence as for the splenius capitis. To also strengthen the part of the muscle that helps bend the head to the side, do the same strengthening exercise with the head bent to the side. Remember to not push the neck muscles too hard.

Bending Sideways (Lateral Flexion)
Primary Mover: Scalene
Opposing Muscle: Scalene on the opposite side

The job of the scalenes is to bend the neck to the same side. Gravity aids this muscle in its job, and you can also use gravity to add resistance.

To Test: Lie on your side on the floor and lift your head and neck slowly toward the ceiling to full pain-free range of motion. Lower down again. Repeat five times.

To Strengthen: Lie on your side on the floor or on a bed with your body aligned with the edge of the bed, arms along your side. Lift your head and neck toward the ceiling. Then lower your head slowly. The muscles are being stretched while contracting (gravity provides resistance). Lift and lower your head three times, lowering it as slowly as you can the last time. *Alternative:* While sitting, reach with one hand over your head to the ear on the other side. Pull your head toward the shoulder of your raised arm while contracting the muscles on the other side to resist the pull.

The Shoulder

Shrugging and Depressing the Shoulders
Primary Mover: Trapezius (upper, middle, and lower parts)
Opposing Muscles: For upper part, Lower trapezius
For middle part, Pectoralis major
For lower part, Upper trapezius

The trapezius's jobs are to lift the shoulders and bend the neck (upper and middle part), to pull the shoulder blade in toward the spine (middle and lower part), and to pull the shoulders back and down (lower part).

To Test: Upper and middle part—raise your shoulders to your ears and lower them five times. Middle and lower part—tests for these are beyond the scope of this book, but since this part of the muscle is used heavily when you lift—for example, as when picking up a heavy wheelbarrow—you can imitate this movement and observe if your trapezius muscle tires from it.

To Strengthen: Upper and middle part—raise and lower your shoulders slowly 10 times. You can also place weights on your shoulders. Middle and lower part—the same as above. However, you strengthen these when you strengthen your middle deltoid, whenever you lift something heavy, and when you do rowing exercises at the gym.

Shrugging the Shoulders (Shoulder Elevation)
Primary Mover: Levator scapulae
Opposing Muscles: Lower trapezius and latissimus dorsi

The levator scapulae's job is to lift the shoulder, help rotate the head to the same side, and help bend the head to the same side.

To Test: Test one side at a time. Place the hand of the side you are testing on the small of your back, which helps isolate the levator scapulae's movement from the trapezius's. Lift and lower your shoulder five times.

To Strengthen: Hold a two-pound weight, one in each hand and perform the same exercise as in the test, holding the weight in the hand of the shoulder you are exercising. Lift and lower three times, lowering very slowly the third time. Repeat this sequence three times.

Pulling the Shoulders Back (Scapular Adduction)
Primary Movers: Rhomboids
Opposing Muscle: Pectoralis major

The job of the rhomboids is to pull the shoulder blades toward the spine and ribs and rotate the shoulder blades downward.

To Test: Hold a two-pound weight in each hand. Lie on your stomach on the floor in a hands-up position. Lift your forearms up toward the ceiling and lower once.

To Strengthen: Using two-pound weights, do the same as above. When lifting your arms, concentrate on only pulling the inner borders of the shoulder blades together (you do not need to lift your arms very far off the floor). Next, move your elbows in the direction of your feet (this rotates the shoulder blades down). Lift, move, and lower three times, lowering slowly the third time. Repeat this sequence three times. You can also strengthen one muscle at a time using the movement in the test.

Bringing the Shoulder Blades away from the Spine (Scapular Abduction)

Primary Mover: Serratus anterior
Opposing Muscles: Rhomboids

The serratus anterior's job is to cement the shoulder blades against the rib cage while bringing the shoulder blades out away from the spine, as occurs in the pushing-up movement of a push-up.

To Test: Stand facing a wall. Extend your arms in front of you at a 90-degree angle (parallel to the floor) and place your hands on the wall. Do a standing push-up slowly in against the wall and back. Repeat five times.

To Strengthen: Same as above. Do three standing push-ups, pushing away from the wall very slowly the third time. When you have gained enough strength, you can start doing the push-ups on the floor. Push-ups on the floor are easier if you bend your knees and work on a soft carpet.

Raising the Arms (Shoulder Flexion, Abduction, and Extension)

Primary Mover: Deltoid (front, middle, and back parts)
Opposing Muscles: For front part, back part of deltoid
For middle part, pectoralis major, latissimus dorsi
For back part, front part of deltoid

The deltoid's jobs are to lift the arm up in front of the body (front part), to lift the arm out to the side and up (middle part), and to lift the arm up behind the body (back part).

To Test: Test each part separately. Front part: Hold a four- or five-pound weight in each hand. Stand or sit on a chair, holding the weight in your hand. Raise your arm in front of you to 90 degrees and slowly lower it down again. Middle part: Hold a five- or six-pound weight in each hand. Extend your arms straight out to the sides to 90 degrees, and slowly lower them back down. Back part: Hold a four- or five-pound weight in each hand. Raise your arms in back of your body and slowly lower them back down.

To Strengthen: Start with a two-pound weight in each hand. Lie on your back on the floor with the weight in your hand. Lift and lower your arm straight up in front of you three times, lowering it very slowly the third time. Repeat this sequence three times.

Rolled-In Shoulders (Flexion, Adduction, and Internal Rotation)

Primary Mover: Pectoralis major
Opposing Muscles: Rhomboids

The pectoralis major's job is to pull the arm in to the side and across the body, and to help raise the arm up in front of the body.

To Test: Hold a two-pound weight in each hand. Lie on your back on the floor in a hands-up position with your elbows bent to 90 degrees, holding the weights in your hands. Slowly raise your arms until your elbows meet and then lower them again slowly.

To Strengthen: Start with a two-pound weight in both hands. Perform the same movement as in the test. Raise and lower your arms three times, lowering them very slowly the third time. Repeat this sequence twice, and after a couple of weeks, increase the repetitions to three.

Working with the Arms behind the Back

Primary Mover: Latissimus dorsi
Opposing Muscles: Upper trapezius, upper part of pectoralis major

The latissimus dorsi's job is to lift the arms backward at the shoulder, to depress the shoulder and bring the arm in, and to rotate the arm inward.

To Test: Hold a four-pound weight in each hand. Stand with the weight in your hand and your arm lifted in front of you to 90 degrees. Bring your arm down toward the floor and continue lifting it up behind your body. Finally, lower it slowly back down to your side. *Also:* Stand with a five-pound weight in your hand. Bending your elbow, bring your arm up behind your body to the small of your back.

To Strengthen: Hold a two-pound weight in each hand. Lie on your stomach on the floor. Lift your arms up behind your body and lower them back down. Do this three times, lowering the arms very slowly the third time. Repeat the sequence three times. Note that this is a very small range of motion.

The Elbow

Bending the Elbow (Flexion)

Primary Mover: Brachioradialis (Note: The biceps is the primary mover of the elbow, but is not included in the key muscles)
Opposing Muscle: Triceps

The job of the brachioradialis is to bend the arm at the elbow and rotate the forearm into a neutral position.

To Test: Use a five-pound weight. Holding the weight in your hand and your forearm in a neutral position (palm toward the thigh), lift your hand to your mouth and lower it slowly.

To Strengthen: Use a two-pound weight. Perform the same motion as in the weakness test above. Lift and lower your arm three times, lowering very slowly the third time. Repeat the sequence three times.

Straightening the Elbow (Extension)

Primary Mover: Triceps
Opposing Muscles: Brachioradilalis, biceps

The job of the triceps is to straighten the arm at the elbow.

To Test: Stand facing a wall with your arms lifted to 90 degrees (shoulder height) and your elbows bent. Position your forearms, elbows, and hands on the wall. Stand with your feet far enough away from the wall that most of your body weight is on your forearms when you lean against the wall. Keeping your hips straight, straighten your arms slowly and then bend them again. Repeat five times.

To Strengthen: Use a two-pound weight. Stand or sit with the weight in your hand. Raise your arm straight up toward the ceiling. Next, bend your arm at the elbow so the hand with the weight moves behind your shoulder in the back. Straighten and bend to lower your arm three times, lowering very slowly the third time. Repeat the sequence three times.

Turning the Forearm Palm Down (Pronation)
Primary Mover: Pronator teres
Opposing Muscle: Supinator

The job of the pronator teres is to rotate the forearm inward, with the hand palm down.

To Test: Use a two-pound weight. Sit on a chair with armrests. Lean your elbow on the armrest with your forearm extending off it. Hold the weight in your hand with your forearm turned inward, palm down. Rotate your forearm up and outward as far as it will go. Then rotate your arm inward and back to the starting position. Repeat five times.

To strengthen: Perform the same motion as above. Rotate and return three times, the third time returning very slowly. Repeat the sequence twice.

Rotating the Forearm Palm Up (Supination)
Primary Mover: Supinator
Opposing Muscle: Pronator teres

The supinator's job is to rotate the forearm outward, turning the hand palm up.

To Test: Use a two-pound weight. Sit on a chair with armrests and lean your elbow on it. Hold the weight in your hand with your forearm turned outward, palm up. Rotate your forearm inward as far as it will go and then rotate it back outward to the starting position. Repeat five times.

To Strengthen: Perform the same motion as above. Rotate and return three times, the third time returning very slowly. Repeat the sequence twice.

The Wrist and Hand

Bending the Hand (Flexion)

Primary Mover: Flexor carpi radialis
Opposing Muscle: Extensor carpi radialis

The job of the flexor carpi radialis is to bend the hand at the wrist.

To Test: Use a two-pound weight. Sit with your elbow leaning on an armrest, the wrist hanging over the edge, and the palm facing up. Holding the weight, bend (flex) your wrist toward you five times.

To Strengthen: Use a two-pound weight. Perform the same motion as above. Bend and straighten three times, the third time straightening very slowly. Repeat the sequence three times.

Lifting the Hand (Extension)

Primary Mover: Extensor carpi ulnaris
Opposing Muscle: Flexor carpi ulnaris

The job of the extensor carpi ulnaris is to lift the hand at the wrist.

To Test: Use a two-pound weight. Sit with your elbow leaning on an armrest and the wrist hanging over the edge, this time with the palm facing down. Holding the weight, lift and lower your hand five times without lifting your forearm.

To Strengthen: Use a two-pound weight. Perform the same motion as in the test above. Lift and lower your hand three times, the third time lowering very slowly. Repeat the sequence three times.

Tensing the Palm

Primary Mover: Palmaris longus
Opposing Muscles: Extensor carpi radialis, extensor carpi ulnaris and extensor digitorum

The job of the palmaris longus is to bend (flex) the wrist and curl the fingers into a claw.

To Test: The same test as for bending the fingers (see below).

To Strengthen: The same exercise as for bending the fingers (see below).

Bending the Fingers (Flexion)
Primary Mover: Flexor digitorum
Opposing Muscle: Extensor digitorum

The flexor digitorum's job is to bend (flex) the fingers and also to help bend the hand at the wrist.

To Test: This requires an unbreakable object such as a raquetball or a can with a diameter of no more than two and a half inches. With your elbow leaning on the table, grip the can or ball. Squeeze your fingers and hand as you lift and set it down five times.

To Strengthen: Perform the same exercise as above. Squeeze as hard as you can. Repeat ten times.

Lifting the Fingers (Extension)
Primary Mover: Extensor digitorum
Opposing Muscle: Flexor digitorum

The extensor digitorum's job is to lift (extend) the fingers and also to help lift the hand at the wrist.

To Test: This requires a thick rubber band or a flat ribbon. Sit sideways at the corner of a table. Place your forearm palm down on the edge of the table so that the base of your fingers is on the edge and the fingers stick out over the edge. Thread the rubber band over the middle knuckles of this hand. Let your free hand hang in the rubber band, providing weight (you do not have to push down—just provide resistance). Lift your fingers up as far as they will go without moving the base of your fingers off the table. Hold for three seconds.

To Strengthen: Begin in the same position as above. Lift your fingers, hold for one second, and lower. Repeat five times (less if the muscles are very weak).

Reaching the Thumb up and out to the Side
(Extension and Abduction)
Primary Movers: Extensor pollicis longus, abductor pollicis
Opposing Muscle: Adductor pollicis

The job of these muscles is to reach the thumb up and out to the side.

To Test: This requires a rubber band. Rest your forearm on a table palm up. Stick your fingers and thumb through the rubber band, placing it over the outer knuckles of your fingers and the end of your thumb. Keep your fingers on the table as you lift the thumb and bring it out to the side as far as it will go. (The rubber band provides resistance.) Slowly bring your thumb back in.

To Strengthen: Perform the same motion as above. Repeat five times.

Moving the Thumb in across the Palm (Adduction)
Primary Movers: Adductor pollicis, opponens pollicis
Opposing Muscles: Extensor pollicis, abductor pollicis

The job of these muscles is to bend the thumb and bring it in across the palm.

To Test: This requires a rubber band. Rest both forearms palms down on a table, one hand's width apart. Reach with your thumbs toward the center and hook them into the rubber band so it loops over the outer knuckle. One thumb at a time, bring your thumb in toward your palm against the resistance of the rubber band.

To Strengthen: Perform the same movement as above. Repeat five times.

The Trunk

Bending Forward (Flexion)
Primary Mover: Rectus abdominis
Opposing Muscle: Erector spinae

The job of the rectus abdominis is to bend the trunk forward.

To Test: Lie on the floor with your knees bent and your feet planted solidly on the floor. Do a sit-up without leaning your hands on the floor. It is easier if you extend your arms straight forward to help you sit up. Repeat three to five times. (It is common to have weak abdominal muscles in need of strengthening.)

To Strengthen: Repeat the sit-up five times. Lower slowly at the last sit-up.

Bending Backward (Extension)
Primary Mover: Erector spinae
Opposing Muscles: Rectus abdominis and iliopsoas

The erector spinae's job is to bend the trunk backward.

To Test: Lie on your stomach on the floor. Raise your upper body slowly as high as it will go, hold, and lower it down again. Repeat five times.

To Strengthen: Perform the same motion as above. Lift your back three times. The third time, hold for three seconds and then lower your body very slowly. Repeat the sequence three times.

Bending the Trunk Sideways (Lateral Flexion)
Primary Mover: Quadratus lumborum
Opposing Muscle: Quadratus lumborum on the other side

The quadratus lumborum's job is to bend the trunk to the same side. You are also testing and strengthening the erector spinae with this exercise.

To Test: Stand up straight and then slowly bend over as far as you can to one side (let one arm slide down your thigh as the other slides up your side). Do the same to the other side. Repeat five times.

To Strengthen: Start this exercise from an upright standing position. Bend very slowly to one side, return to the straight position with equally slow movements. Repeat five times on the same side. Then repeat the entire exercise on the other side.

The Hip

Bending the Hip (Flexion)
Primary Mover: Iliopsoas

Opposing Muscles: Gluteus maximus and hamstrings

The job of the iliopsoas is to bend the body at the hip, as in lifting the thigh toward the body.

To Test: In a standing position, holding onto something for support, lift your knee toward your body five times.

To Strengthen: Perform the same exercise as above, the fifth time lowering your leg slowly. Repeat the sequence three times.

Straightening the Hip (Extension)
Primary Movers: Gluteus maximus and hamstrings
Opposing muscles: Iliopsoas and rectus femoris (one of the quads)

The job of the gluteus maximus is to straighten the hip.

To Test: This requires a chair. Sit on the chair and raise yourself to a standing position, then lower yourself slowly back to a seated position. Repeat five times.

To Strengthen: Perform the same activity as above. Raise and lower yourself three times, the third time lowering yourself very slowly. Repeat this sequence three times.

Rotating the Leg Outward (External Rotation)
Primary Mover: Piriformis
Opposing Muscles: Gluteus minimus (not a key muscle), gluteus medius—front part, and tensor fasciae latae

The job of the piriformis is to rotate the hip out to the side.

To Test: Stand on the leg that you are not testing, holding onto something for support—for example, the back of a chair. Use this for balance, but do not put weight on your hand. Keep your free hand on the hipbone in front to feel the muscle move. Lift the foot of the leg you are testing slightly off the floor and rotate the thigh outward as far as it will go 10 times.

To Strengthen: This time, to add the effect of gravity, lie on the floor on the side you are not testing. Bend your knee a little and rotate your thigh and knee outward. Repeat 10 times. You can also sit on a bench with a

weight tied to your ankle and rotate your thigh outward with the knee
bent.

Pulling the Legs Together (Adduction)

Primary Movers: The adductors
Opposing Muscle: Gluteus medius

The job of the adductors is to bring the thighs together and help bend the
hip forward.

To Test: This requires a low chair. Lie on your side. Place your upper foot
on the seat of the chair. Lift the leg on the floor up to the other leg. Lift and
lower your leg three times.

To Strengthen: Do the same as above. This time, lower the leg very slowly after the third lift. Repeat this sequence three times. You can add resistance by tying a weight to your ankle.

Moving the Thighs Apart (Abduction)

Primary Mover: Gluteus medius
Opposing Muscles: Adductors

The job of the gluteus medius is to move the thigh out to the side and also
to rotate the thigh inward (front part).

To Test: Stand on the leg you are testing with your hands on your hips.
Lift the other leg and bring the foot behind the leg you are standing on.
The hip you are standing on will naturally tilt slightly up, but try to keep
things as level as you can. Stand like this for one minute. It will not seem as
if the muscle is doing its job, but it is in fact contracting while being
stretched. In daily life, this muscle is worked if you tend to put your weight
on one leg for an extended period of time, as it maintains alignment of the
hip so it does not sag on one side.

To Strengthen: Lie on your side. Lift your leg up as far as it will go and
then lower it. Lift and lower the leg three times, the third time lowering it
very slowly. Repeat this sequence three times. When you get stronger, you
can add a weight to your leg (two pounds or more, depending on your
strength).

The following muscle moves both the hip and the knee, but it is not the primary mover for either:

Muscle: Tensor fasciae latae
Opposing muscle: Gluteus maximus

The tensor fasciae latae's job is to bend (flex) the hip, to move the thigh out to the side, and to rotate the thigh inward.

To Test: Lie on your side. Rotate your thigh inward, lift it up as far as it will go, and then lower it. Rotate, lift, and lower your leg three times.

To Strengthen: Do the same as above, but this time rotate, lift, and lower your leg three times, the third time lowering it very slowly. Repeat this sequence three times. To increase strength, tie a weight (two or four pounds) on your lower leg.

The Knee

Bending the Knee (Flexion)
Primary Movers: Hamstrings
Opposing Muscles: Quadriceps

The job of the hamstrings is to bend the knee and straighten the hip.

To Test: Use a four-pound or heavier weight and tie it on your foot. While standing, lift your lower leg, bringing your heel to your buttocks. Repeat three times.

To Strengthen: Do the same as above. This time lift and lower your lower leg three times, the third time lowering it very slowly. Repeat this sequence three times.

Straightening the Knee (Extension)
Primary Movers: Quadriceps
Opposing Muscles: Hamstrings

The job of the quadriceps is to straighten the knee and also to bend the hip (only one of the quads does this—the rectus femoris).

To Test: From a standing position, bend your knees and squat about halfway down to the floor. Rise back up slowly. Repeat five times.

To Strengthen: You can do this with or without weights. Sit on a chair. Lift your lower leg to straighten the knee and then lower it back down. Lift and lower three times, the third time lowering the leg very slowly. Repeat the sequence five times.

The Foot

Bending the Foot Down—Pointing the Toes (Plantar Flexion)
Primary Movers: Calf muscles
Opposing Muscle: Tibialis anterior

The job of the calf muscles is to bend the foot down, as in pointing the foot.

To Test: Stand balanced on a stair with your heel hanging off the step. Rise up on your toes as high as you can, keeping your knees straight and without leaning to the side. Lower your heels and repeat 10 times.

To Strengthen: Do the same as above. Rise and lower three times, the third time lowering your heels very slowly. Repeat this sequence three times. To increase the resistance, you can put weights on your shoulders.

Bending the Foot Up (Dorsiflexion)
Primary Mover: Tibialis anterior
Opposing Muscles: Calf muscles

The tibialis anterior's job is to bend the foot up.

To Test: Use a four-pound weight. Sitting on a bench with your feet dangling, put the weight on your toes (the homemade weight works very well when you leave a space between the cans so it lies on your foot). Lift your toes toward your shin and lower 10 times.

To Strengthen: Use a four-pound weight. Do the same motion as in the test above, with a weight on your foot. Repeat 10 times. After the 5th and 10th lifts, lower your foot slowly.

Turning the Sole of the Foot out to the Side (Eversion)
Primary Mover: Peroneus
Opposing Muscle: Tibialis anterior

The job of the peroneus is to turn the sole of the foot outward to the side and also to help bend the foot down, as in pointing your foot.

To Test: Use a four-pound weight. Tie it to your foot. Lie on the floor with your leg raised and your foot parallel to the floor. Turn the sole of your foot outward first and then point your foot. Repeat five times.

To Strengthen: Use a four-pound weight. Do the same as above. Repeat 10 times. After the 5th and 10th times, turn the sole of the foot inward and lower your toes very slowly.

Lifting the Toes (Extension)
Primary Movers: Extensor digitorum longus and extensor hallucis longus
Opposing Muscle: Flexor hallucis longus

The job of these muscles is to lift the toes and to help bend the foot up with the toes toward your shin.

To Test: While standing with both feet on the floor, slowly lift your toes, including the big toe, up from the floor as far as they go. Repeat 10 times.

To Strengthen: While standing or sitting, put your toes under a surface that will not move (for example, the bottom of a couch). Against this resistance, attempt to lift your toes. Repeat 10 times.

Appendix 1: Quick Reference for Locating Key Muscles

Note: Only the 36 muscles described in this book are listed here.

THE NECK
Front: Sternocleidomastoid (SCM) muscle, scalenes
Back: Trapezius—upper part, splenii, levator scapulae
Sides: Scalenes, levator scapulae

THE SHOULDER
Front: Front of the deltoid, pectoralis major
Back: Back of the deltoid, trapezius—upper and middle part, triceps
Sides: Side of the deltoid

THE UPPER TRUNK
Front: Pectoralis major, serratus anterior
Back: Trapezius—middle part, rhomboids, erector spinae
Side: Serratus anterior

THE UPPER ARM
Front: Biceps (not a key muscle), brachioradialis (starts $1/3$ down)
Back: Triceps
Side: Triceps

THE FOREARM
(with Palms Facing Each Other)
Top: Brachioradialis
Inside: Flexor carpi ulnaris, palmaris longus, flexor digitorum, pronator teres
Outside: Extensor carpi radialis, extensor digitorum, supinator, extensor pollicis longus

THE HAND

Palm: Palmaris longus, flexor digitorum, adductor pollicis
Back: Extensor digitorum, extensor carpi radialis

THE TRUNK

Back: Erector spinae, quadratus lumborum, latissimus dorsi, trapezius—lower part
Front: Rectus abdominis, iliopsoas
Side: Serratus anterior

THE HIP

Front: Iliopsoas, rectus abdominis
Back: Gluteus maximus, quadratus lumborum, piriformis, erector spinae, latissimus dorsi
Side: Gluteus maximus, gluteus medius, piriformis, tensor fasciae latae

THE THIGH

Front: Quadriceps
Back: Hamstrings
Inside: Adductors
Outside: Tensor fasciae latae

THE LOWER LEG

Front: Tibialis anterior, extensor digitorum, extensor hallucis longus
Back: Calf muscles
Outside: Peroneus
Inside: Calf muscles

THE FOOT

Top: Extensor hallicus longus, tibialis anterior
Bottom: Peroneus, tibialis anterior

Appendix 2: Charts for Recording Your Progress

TEST RESULTS

Range	N (Normal)	T (Tight)	TT (Very tight)	L (Left side)	R (Right side)	L/R (Both sides)	P (Pain)	NP (No pain)
Neck								
Home test 1								
Home test 2								
Home test 3								
Home test 4								
Shoulder								
Home test 1								
Home test 2								
Home test 3								
Home test 4								
Home test 5								
Home test 6								
Home test 7								
Home test 8								
Home test 9								
Elbow								
Home test 1								
Home test 2								
Home test 3								
Home test 4								
Hand and Wrist								
Home test 1								
Home test 2								
Home test 3								
Home test 5								
Home test 6								
Home test 7								
Home test 8								

Range	N (Normal)	T (Tight)	TT (Very tight)	L (Left side)	R (Right side)	L/R (Both sides)	P (Pain)	NP (No pain)
Trunk								
Home test 1								
Home test 2								
Home test 3								
Home test 4								
Hip and Thigh								
Home test 1								
Home test 2								
Home test 3								
Home test 4								
Home test 5								
Home test 6								
Home test 7								
Home test 8								
Home test 9								
Knee								
Home test 1								
Home test 2								
Ankle								
Home test 1								
Home test 2								

PAIN DIAGRAM

Use this entire page to draw the outlines of a body, seen from the front and the back. Mark with a star the exact areas of your body that are most sore and painful.

Front   *Back*

Glossary

abuse of a muscle   Any trauma, lack of use, misuse, overuse, or lack of sufficient blood supply and nerve stimulus

active stretch   The stretch that takes place when you consciously contract some muscles in order to stretch others

arteries   The blood vessels that transport blood from the heart to all tissue in the body

assisting muscle   A muscle whose function is to assist another muscle in carrying out its job

beginning tendon   The attachment site (origin) of a muscle

blood vessel constriction   Narrowing that takes place when the diameter of a blood vessel decreases, thereby causing less blood to flow to tissues, organs, and muscles

blood vessel dilation   Opening that takes place when the diameter of a blood vessel increases, causing more blood to flow to tissues, organs, and muscles

bony landmarks   The bony bumps that a muscle's tendons attach to

capillaries   The tiny blood vessels in tissues, organs, and muscles that allow nutrients and waste products to be exchanged through their thin walls

cartilage   The tissue that covers the surface of the bones at the site of a joint

collagen   A fibrous, insoluble protein, found in connective tissue, that has the ability to yield gelatin and tissue fibers

connective tissue   Tissue made of collagen fibers that pervades, supports, and binds together other structures in the body

edema   An excess accumulation of fluid found in the connective tissue

ending tendon   The attachment site (insertion) of a muscle

fascia   A sheet of connective tissue that covers whole muscles, individual muscle fibers, and bundles of fibers

goniometer   A plastic instrument with two arms, one that is fixed and one that moves, joined to form an angle, used to measure the range of motion at a joint

homeostasis   The maintenance of stable internal physiological status—a pain-free balance between substances in the body

hypertonic   Excessive tone or tension in a muscle

inflammation   A local response to cellular injury that causes dilation of the capillaries, redness, heat, and/or swelling as part of the natural process of repair

involuntary muscles   The muscles that you cannot control (smooth muscles); for example, the muscles surrounding the blood vessels that cause constriction or dilation (*see also* Voluntary muscles)

ischemia   Tissue anemia arising from a lack of oxygen caused by obstruction of arterial blood flow to the tissue, resulting in lack of vigor and weakness

length monitor   Sensory organs in a muscle that consist of small fibers richly supplied with nerve fibers, located in the muscle fibers, enclosed in connective tissue, and particularly sensitive to stretch

ligament   Connective tissue that attaches a bone to another bone

metabolism   The chemical processes and changes that occur in living cells

muscle belly   The soft, fleshy part of the muscle that is located between the two tendon sites

muscle/tendon junction   The exact spot where the muscle fibers end and the tendon fibers begin

nociceptors   *See* Pain receptors

opposing muscle   A muscle whose function is to perform the opposite job of another muscle

pain receptors   Nerve endings (nociceptors) in the tissue that are aggravated when chemicals in the tissue exceed an acceptable level

passive stretch   A stretch that is caused not by actively contracting a muscle, but by passively pulling the muscle into a stretched position

peripheral nerve   A nerve outside the central nervous system (spine and brain)

primary mover   A muscle primarily responsible for movement at a joint

postural muscle   A muscle that holds your body upright against the force of gravity, such as your back and neck muscles but not your finger muscles

range of motion   The range of movement available at a joint, which can be limited by tight or weak muscles

resting length of a muscle   Describes a muscle that is neither contracted nor stretched, but is between the two positions

scar tissue   New connective tissue produced at the site of an injury to repair the wound caused by that injury

standard range   The range of motion at a joint established by medical doctors and physical therapists as the minimum range necessary for healthy functioning

stretch reflex   A spinal reflex involving reflexive contraction of muscle fibers in response to stretching, regulated by the length monitors

tendon   The connective tissue that attaches a muscle to the bone

tendon attachment site   The exact location where the tendon fibers attach on the bone

tension monitors   The sensory organs within a tendon, located where the muscle fibers meet the tendon fibers, that provide information about muscle tension

veins   The blood vessels that transport blood from the tissue back to the lungs

voluntary muscles   The muscles in the body (skeletal muscles) that are under your conscious control (*see also* Involuntary muscles)

waste products   The by-products of vital activity in the muscles

Bibliography

Berne, Robert M., and Matthew N. Levy. *Cardiovascular Physiology.* St. Louis: Mosby, 1997.

Cailliet, Rene. *Soft Tissue Pain and Disability.* Philadelphia: F. A. Davis Company, 1996.

Calais-German, Blandine. *Anatomy of Movement.* Seattle: Eastland Press, 1996.

Cassvan, Arminius, et al. *Cumulative Trauma Disorders.* Boston: Butterworth-Heinemann, 1997.

Evjenth, Olaf, and Jern Hamberg. *Autostretching.* Alfta, Sweden: Alfta Rehab Forlag, 1989.

Floyd, R. T., and Clem W. Thompson. *Manual of Structural Kinesiology.* St. Louis: Mosby, 1994.

Fritz, Sandy, Kathleen Maison Paholsky, and M. James Grosenbach. *Soft Tissue and Movement Therapies.* St. Louis: Mosby, 1999.

Hislop, Helen J., et al. *Daniels and Worthingham's Muscle Testing.* London: W. B. Saunders, 1995.

Hoppenfeldt, Stanley. *Physical Examination of the Spine and Extremities.* Norwalk, Conn.: Appleton & Lange, 1976.

Husum, Hans, et al. *War Surgery: Field Manual.* Malaysia: Third World Network, 1995.

Jones, David, et al. *Skeletal Muscle in Health and Disease.* Manchester, U.K.: Manchester University Press, 1990.

Jozsa, Laszlo G., et al. *Human Tendons—Anatomy, Physiology and Pathology.* Champaign, Ill.: Human Kinetics, 1997.

Lederman, Eyal. *Fundamentals of Manual Therapy.* New York: Churchill Livingstone, 1997.

Levick, J. R. *An Introduction to Cardiovascular Physiology.* Oxford: Butterworth-Heinemann, 1998.

Lippert, Lynn S. *Clinical Kinesiology for Physical Therapist Assistants.* Philadelphia: F. A. Davis Company, 1994.

Palmer, Lynn, and Marcia Epler. *Clinical Assessment Procedures in Physical Therapy.* Philadelphia: J. B. Lippincott Company, 1990.

Pitt-Brook, J., et al. *Rehabilitation of Movement.* London: W. B. Saunders, 1998.

Robergs, Robert A., and Scott O. Roberts. *Exercise Physiology.* St. Louis: Mosby, 1997.

Travell, Janet, et al. *Myofascial Pain and Dysfunction.* Philadelphia: Lippincott Williams & Wilkins, 1979.

Wittink, Harriet, and Theresa Hoskins Michel. *Chronic Pain Management for Physical Therapists.* Boston: Butterworth-Heinemann, 1997.

Index

About the Author

Elisabeth Aaslid is a writer, translator, and teacher. The challenge of attempting to resolve recurring muscle pain conditions she and her family experienced led her to study physiology and anatomy for several years while working with experts in the fields of physical and massage therapy. During this time she developed her skills and pioneering work in understanding and relieving muscle pain.

Elisabeth grew up in a health-and-fitness-focused environment in a family of doctors in Oslo, Norway, and has since resided in Britain, Norway, Switzerland, and, for the last 15 years, the United States. She is a graduate of the University of Oslo and Rose Bruford College, London, with coursework in playwriting at the University of Washington. Her wide range of writing includes several plays, one of which was performed in Seattle in 1994. She is currently teaching business communications at the University of Washington, teaching classes and conducting workshops on understanding and healing muscle pain at Applied Health & Body Works in Seattle, as well as providing such education through her Internet Web site.

Kate A. Schultz, P.T., has dealt extensively with acute muscular pain conditions in her work as a physical therapist in lower back, hospital, and general pediatrics clinics. Her special focus is manual muscle testing and range of motion testing. She is a graduate in physical therapy from the University of Iowa and studied zoology, kinesiology, and physical education at Iowa State University. Kate has acted as a collaborator on this book.